T0144638

BASIC HEALTH
PUBLICATIONS
USER'S GUIDE

TO
COENZYME
Q10

Don't Be a Dummy.
Become an Expert on
What Coenzyme Q10
Can Do for Your
Health.

MARTIN ZUCKER
JACK CHALLEM Series Editor

The information contained in this book is based upon the research and personal and professional experiences of the author. It is not intended as a substitute for consulting with your physician or other health care provider. Any attempt to diagnose and treat an illness should be done under the direction of a health care professional.

The publisher does not advocate the use of any particular health care protocol but believes the information in this book should be available to the public. The publisher and author are not responsible for any adverse effects or consequences resulting from the use of the suggestions, preparations, or procedures discussed in this book. Should the reader have any questions concerning the appropriateness of any procedures or preparation mentioned, the author and the publisher strongly suggest consulting a professional health care advisor.

Series Editor: Jack Challem
Editor: Roberta W. Waddell
Typesetter: Gary A. Rosenberg
Series Cover Designer: Mike Stromberg

Basic Health Publications User's Guides are published by Basic Health Publications, Inc.
www.basichealthpub.com

ISBN: 978-1-59120-010-9 (Pbk.)
ISBN: 978-1-68162-848-6 (Hardcover)

CONTENTS

INTRODUCTION

You are the sum of your cellular parts—all several hundred trillion cells. And how you feel and function depends on how they feel and function. And how they feel and function has a lot to do with coenzyme Q_{10}, better known as CoQ_{10}, a vitaminlike substance produced throughout your body. Without this substance, your cells—and thus, *you*—couldn't survive.

For starters, CoQ_{10} is a fundamental ingredient in the energy production that keeps those trillions of cells running smoothly. A shortage of CoQ_{10} translates into an energy crunch, with you and your cells running on weak batteries.

Unfortunately, that situation describes a lot of people, many of whom are outright deficient. Low levels of CoQ_{10} generate a negative impact on health and, very likely, the aging process itself.

Besides generating energy, CoQ_{10} is one of the body's most powerful antioxidants. It protects you against free radicals, the destructive molecular fragments that cause accelerated aging and degenerative diseases. And, according to exciting new research, CoQ_{10} also activates certain genes in a way that appears to strengthen you against disease and rejuvenate your body.

Sadly, most doctors either haven't heard of CoQ_{10} or just ignore its importance. That's a tragedy because simply increasing the level of CoQ_{10} in the body pays off with big health, energy, and therapeutic dividends.

Fortunately, CoQ_{10} is available as a nutritional

supplement. It's a natural copy of what your body makes, and it's wonderfully safe to take. Unlike pharmaceutical drugs, you don't develop bad side effects from taking it. Moreover, you don't need a prescription. You can buy it in health food stores just as you would vitamin C, gingko biloba, or any other supplement.

Since the 1960s, scientists in Japan, Europe, Australia, India, and the United States have been studying the healing impact of CoQ_{10}, primarily on cardiovascular conditions. But during the last decade, research has expanded dynamically into many age-related diseases, including baffling brain disorders, as well as the aging process itself.

To date, there have been more than four thousand scientific studies and eleven international conferences dedicated to CoQ_{10}. Yet researchers feel they have only scratched the surface in their understanding of CoQ_{10}'s formidable functions and how supplementation may contribute to better health. What's known to date distinguishes CoQ_{10} as a healing superstar and lifesaver.

Continuing research promises much more good news. In laboratories and clinics worldwide, researchers and doctors are discovering major therapeutic and preventive uses for CoQ_{10}. In this book, you'll learn about the benefits and promise of CoQ_{10}, including:

- Disease prevention and slowing down the aging process in the body;

- Significant help for patients with heart disease;

- Reduction of mild to moderate hypertension;

- More energy, strength, and vitality, even for older people;

- Fortification of the immune system against illness, including cancer;

- Counteracting the adverse effects of cholesterol-lowering drugs;

- Improvement of nervous system and brain disorders; and

- Protection against gum disease, a condition affecting most adults.

These are all major considerations for individuals interested in optimum health and optimum lifespan. As you read on you will learn how CoQ_{10} contributes to both.

CHAPTER 1

An Amazing Molecule "Born" in a Refrigerator

Back in 1957, Fred Crane, Ph.D., was a young research biochemist and assistant professor working at the University of Wisconsin's Enzyme Institute. He and his colleagues were investigating the biochemical sequence involved in cellular energy production.

Crane, now seventy-six years old and retired, recalls, "we could partly put the sequence together, but something was missing in our understanding of these molecular events. I was assigned the job to find the missing link."

The researchers were working with beef-heart mitochondria. Mitochondria are where energy is produced inside cells. You will be hearing a lot about them in this book.

Mitochondria

Mitochondria are organelles—microscopic organs—within cells where oxygen and the derivatives of the food you eat are mixed to produce energy. Think of the mitochondria as the "power plants" that generate the energy to operate individual cells.

Mitochondria, present in both animal and plant cells, are center stage for the activity of CoQ_{10}. But Crane and his team didn't know it at the time. In fact, no scientist had ever heard of CoQ_{10}.

Extracurricular Research Pays Off

On weekends, Crane liked to return to the laboratory and continue his scientific sleuthing. At one point he began examining cauliflower mitochondria.

"This wasn't part of the program, but I always enjoyed variety, doing something different," he says. "So I chopped up the cauliflower, centrifuged the mush, and separated out the mitochondria. On Monday mornings, when my colleagues returned to the lab, they would complain that I was stinking up the place with cauliflower."

Smell aside, Crane's extracurricular research led to pay dirt. He first discovered carotenes (pigments) in the cauliflower mitochondria. He thought these could be the sought-after missing link. Turning back to beef hearts, he found a small amount of carotenes, but a large mass of yellowish substance that had different properties. He collected the material and put it aside in the lab's refrigerator while he continued studying the carotenes.

"One day I looked back in the fridge," he recalls, "and there was this tube full of the other stuff which had formed big yellow crystals. I thought maybe it might be good for something."

From Beef Hearts to the Nobel Prize

Measuring the material with a technique called light-absorption spectrum, Crane determined that it was a quinone—a family of organic compounds that he knew to have properties related to energy conversion.

Looking for confirmation, he sent off a sample of the yellow stuff to Karl Folkers, Ph.D., a leading biochemist at Merck, Sharpe, and Dohme Laboratories in New Jersey. Folkers' analysis showed that the substance was indeed a quinone, and just in case you are interested, he identified its chemical structure as 2,3, dimethoxy-5-methyl-6-decaprenyl-1,4-benzoquinone. It was a relatively large, worm-shaped molecule.

Other biochemists would call it ubiquinone because the molecule was found to be ubiquitous—widespread in living organisms.

Indeed, it turned out to be the missing link, and a major link at that.

Some years later, in 1978, British biochemist Peter Mitchell, Ph.D., would earn the Nobel Prize in chemistry for describing the complicated and exquisite process of cellular power production. And there, smack in the middle of that process, would be CoQ_{10}.

Birth of a CoQ_{10} Champion

But back in 1958, Crane's shipment of yellow stuff set off a flurry of scientific investigation at the Merck lab. Folkers and his colleagues dug into it with relish. They soon learned how to synthesize the compound, which they named coenzyme Q_{10} (CoQ_{10} for short). A coenzyme is a substance like a vitamin that contributes to essential chemical reactions, and in the case of CoQ_{10}, it contributes to "bioenergetics," the process of cellular energy production.

Folkers left Merck in 1963 to become president of Stanford Research Institute, a position he held for five years. Then, for the next thirty years, he served as research professor of chemistry, and later as director of the Institute for Biomedical Research at the University of Texas in Austin.

Folkers had been smitten by CoQ_{10}. And until his death in 1997 at age ninety-one, he ardently conducted and encouraged research on the basic biochemistry and clinical applications of CoQ_{10}.

Absolutely Essential for Life

In 1972, along with Italian researcher Gian Paolo Littarru, M.D., Folkers first determined there was a deficiency of CoQ_{10} in heart disease. This original research led to numerous studies showing major therapeutic benefits for heart patients supplemented with CoQ_{10}. (In Chapter 5 you can read more about the great connection to heart health.)

For years, much of the research and the clinical uses of CoQ_{10} centered on the heart and cardiovascular system. But more recently, scientists have looked beyond the heart and found promising uses for it against cancer, muscle, and brain disorders, as well as its intriguing potential as an "antiaging" factor.

The mounting reports from researchers worldwide validate Folkers' belief that medical science would come to recognize many important benefits for CoQ_{10}. He repeatedly told interviewers that "every life function requires biochemical energy and CoQ_{10} is a major mechanism in the process. It is absolutely essential for life."

For his years of outstanding research, Folkers received many honors, including presidential science awards from Harry Truman in 1948 and George Bush in 1990.

Your Body Makes CoQ_{10}, But . . .

Almost every cell in the body produces CoQ_{10}, yet many people are deficient in CoQ_{10}. Here are five reasons why:

Reason No. 1: Diet

It takes a number of key ingredients for your body to synthesize, or make, CoQ_{10}. The recipe calls for the amino acid tyrosine and at least seven vitamins (B_2, B_3, B_6, folic acid, B_{12}, C, pantothenic acid).

According to Folkers, "The problem is that people in general eat poorly, and don't get an adequate level of good nutrients, so they often fail to produce enough."

This assessment fits right in with current nutritional surveys, which consistently find a large percentage of people deficient in essential vitamins and minerals.

Take vitamin B_6, for example, one of the critical ingredients in the CoQ_{10} recipe. If you look at any list of common deficiencies, you'll find B_6 a regular entry. The vitamin is particularly low among older people and those eating a diet high in refined carbohydrates and low in vegetables and fruits. One study specifically designed to look at this connection did indeed determine that the customary intake of vitamin B_6 doesn't support an optimum production of CoQ_{10}.

You can extract some CoQ_{10} directly from the food you eat. But that depends on what you eat. CoQ_{10} is naturally present in small quantities in many foods. The best sources are organ meats such as heart, kidney, and liver, as well as mackerel, peanuts, salmon, sardines, and soy oil—foods we tend not to eat a lot.

Just to obtain the equivalent of a 30-mg supplement, you would have to eat one pound of sardines, two pounds of beef, or two and one-half pounds of peanuts. Thirty milligrams may be fine for general health maintenance, but it isn't nearly enough to produce therapeutic benefits against disease.

Cardiologist Peter Langsjoen, M.D., of Tyler, Texas, has used CoQ_{10} for his patients longer than any other physician in the country. He says that even by eating a lot of fish you can probably only consume the equivalent of 5–10 mg a day.

"That's what the average Dane gets in a diet high in fish," he says. "But without the fish it is likely you will only get 3 to 5 mg. The key is fish. It's loaded with CoQ_{10}. Also beef, chicken, and pork hearts . . . but nobody eats them."

Langsjoen says his new patients are typically deficient. That's also the experience of Stephen T. Sinatra, M.D., a cardiologist in Manchester, Connecticut, who became so impressed with CoQ_{10} that he wrote a book about it: *The Coenzyme Q_{10} Phenomenon* (Keats Publishing, 1998).

"I regularly do blood levels of CoQ_{10} and find that new patients are low," he says. "I believe there are significant deficiencies in the population."

Reason No. 2: The Aging Factor

The body's production of CoQ_{10} slows down with age. Scientists say it starts happening after the age of twenty, with a more accelerated drop after forty.

"Production kind of poops out," says CoQ_{10} discoverer Fred Crane. "And the most obvious place where CoQ_{10} works is in the mitochondria. So, if you don't have enough, then you might not produce energy as well in your cells. This may help to explain why older people slow down."

Reason No. 3: Cholesterol Drugs

The pharmaceutical industry is vigorously promoting cholesterol-lowering drugs (statins), even among healthy people as a preventive agent, yet this class of pharmaceuticals has a dark side that few people know about. Research shows these drugs interfere with CoQ_{10} production in the body.

This is a major problem that will be discussed in detail in Chapter 5.

Reason No. 4: Extreme Physical Exertion

Regular moderate exercise is thought to stimulate the body's production of CoQ_{10}. However, experts say that exhaustive and prolonged exercise depletes CoQ_{10}. That's because the body needs more of it to fuel the increased activity.

At risk are high performance athletes as well as weekend-warrior types who go out and cycle 100 miles or run 20 miles on a weekend.

"They burn up a tremendous amount of CoQ_{10}, and other nutrients necessary for CoQ_{10} production," says Langsjoen. "And if they are not replacing these factors in their diet, they may be hurting themselves."

The cardiologist cites the case of a patient fresh from Navy Seal training who had heart muscle weakness. "These are very tough and fit people who go through incredibly exhausting training," Langsjoen says. "They have a grinding schedule, and then to top it off, go days without rest.

"I have seen heart muscle weakness in many obsessive, compulsive joggers who essentially run themselves down. I wonder if that is what happened with the Navy Seal. It's not proven, but I think a deficiency state is created. The end result is a dilated heart."

Reason No. 5: Hyperthyroidism

An overactive thyroid gland—hyperthyroidism—raises the level of thyroid hormone in the body. This can cause such typical signs as anxiety, bulging of the eyes, fast or irregular heart rhythms, irritability, muscle weakness, and weight loss.

Too much thyroid hormone accelerates metabolism. One of the less recognized consequences of this is the drain put on the body's CoQ_{10} supply, which can, in turn, deplete CoQ_{10} and cause additional problems.

"The heart is usually a primary target," says Sinatra. "Not only arrhythmias, but even heart failure may result. I have seen the connection to heart failure in patients who were not previously diagnosed with overactive thyroid and who didn't have the usual hyperthyroid symptoms."

Sinatra suggests that patients with thyroid irregularities, and particularly with excess thyroid hormone, should be on supplemental CoQ_{10}.

CHAPTER 2

THE GREAT ENERGIZER

Y ou probably know somebody like one of my relatives (who shall remain anonymous). After a typical workday, he would sit back in his living room easy chair and do the typical couch-potato thing: watch TV for a couple of hours and then doze off. That was his pattern before he began taking CoQ_{10}.

"Now," he says, "I go out more with my wife, have gotten involved in more activities, and don't feel as bone tired as I used to. My energy level has really improved. I feel a whole lot younger."

At fifty-two, my relative had become concerned about learning new tasks at his job and about what he felt was increasing forgetfulness. He thought he might be developing Alzheimer's disease.

"But since taking CoQ_{10}, I have found that I can again concentrate and learn as well as when I was younger," he confided. "I really believe this CoQ_{10} stuff has given me a lot of physical and mental energy back."

Such comments are typical of CoQ_{10} users and even of physicians who recommend CoQ_{10} supplementation to patients.

Your Energy Level Depends on Your Cells

You eat, drink, and breathe. Deep down in the mitochondria of your cells the ingredients of those fundamental actions are converted into the energy to unleash countless thoughts, secretions, nerve impulses, and muscle contractions.

The mitochondria, as you will remember from

Chapter 1, are the microscopic "power plants" in your cells where the wondrous biochemical process called "bioenergetics" goes on endlessly during a lifetime.

Inside these rod- or round-shaped dynamos is an inner sanctum of membrane folds projecting inward from the outer membrane. An extremely complex sequence of chemical reactions takes place in these membranes involving enzymes, protons, electrons, and electrical charges.

For the sake of simplicity, think of a cell gathering in oxygen, along with sugars and fatty acids from food, and dispatching them to the mitochondria. There, the raw materials are processed by enzymes to produce a substance called adenosine triphosphate, or ATP for short. ATP acts like a high-octane fuel to stoke virtually all the cells in the body.

> **Enzymes**
> *Specialized proteins that make possible biochemical reactions. Without them, our body chemistry would not occur, and life would not exist. The names of enzymes end in "ase."*

Electrons extracted from the food are utilized to make ATP. CoQ_{10} molecules carry out a starring role in this process by shuttling electrons back and forth between enzymes. This, according to Karl Folkers, is the primary function of CoQ_{10} in the body.

The arrangement inside the mitochondria is like a precision assembly line. Raw materials come in at one end. ATP molecules come out the other.

Works Like a Car Engine

You can also think of this process in terms of a car engine. It takes oxygen and gasoline, and a spark, to create the energy to drive the pistons to turn the crankshaft to move the wheels.

Just as engine problems can cause a car to malfunction or operate feebly, problems with mitochondria can cause similar trouble in the body.

The cells in the body each contain between five hundred and two thousand mitochondria. When they don't function properly, an "energy crisis" develops. Faltering energy production in individual cells initiates a cascade of disorder and inefficiency throughout the body. Over time, the damage from energy shortfall spreads to tissues and organ systems.

Brain, heart, and muscle cells, the heaviest consumers of energy, start to struggle. They stop performing well. They fail to carry out their basic functions. If enough vitality and function is lost, affected cells commit suicide. Tissues begin to degenerate.

CoQ_{10} Deficiency Spells Trouble

Think about it. Cells need energy to perform all the specialized things they do for the body, such as producing enzymes, hormones, muscle contractions, and nerve impulses, fighting off bacteria and viruses, or breaking down food with acids. Cells also have to carry out basic household chores, such as nourishing themselves and getting rid of waste products. And cells also have to reproduce—we started, after all, from one fertilized egg cell. All this requires energy.

Cardiologist Stephen Sinatra sums it up this way: "Without adequate energy the cells become inefficient, lackluster, and vulnerable to disease and toxic buildup. When a deficiency of CoQ_{10} exists, the cellular 'engines' misfire and, over time, they may eventually fail or even die. The bioenergetics of a failing heart or a failing immune system will inevitably lead to the weakening of all the natural defenses against disease and premature aging."

That's how vital CoQ_{10} is to your cells and, ultimately, to you. And that's why supplementation can make a big difference in energy for so many people. Remember, we lose some of our ability to produce CoQ_{10} as we get older, so don't be caught short.

CHAPTER 3

THE GREAT ANTIOXIDANT

When a nuclear bomb explodes, the blast of powerful radiation triggers a firestorm of "free radicals" that virtually wipes out everything in its path. Free radicals are not showers of shrapnel. Rather they are runaway electrons that create chain reactions of destruction at the atomic level.

There are no atomic bombs in the cells of our body, but chain reactions instigated by electrons go on everywhere and all the time.

As we have seen, our cells utilize oxygen atoms to produce energy in the mitochondria. One byproduct of this normal process is the constant creation of a huge number of free radicals. This poses a threat not only to the mitochondria but also to the rest of the cell.

Free radicals are simply "free" electrons that have broken loose from their attachments to the nuclei of oxygen atoms during the energy process. Electrons like company, so they seek other electrons to pair up with. This activity, repeated countless times in countless cells, sets off a chain reaction of damage that starts with adjacent atoms and molecules. Over time, it engulfs tissues and eventually organ systems.

This domino effect, first theorized more than thirty years ago by Denham Harman, M.D., Ph.D., a University of Nebraska researcher, is the most widely accepted scientific explanation for aging. His free radical theory of aging holds that free radicals are causal factors in nearly every known disease, as well as the aging process itself.

Terrorists inside Our Bodies

Free radicals are like terrorists inside our bodies. They attack DNA, leading to dysfunction, mutation, and cancer. They attack enzymes and proteins, causing mayhem in normal cell activities. They attack cell membranes.

In the cells that line our blood vessels, this can lead to hardening and thickening of the arteries and eventually to heart attacks and strokes. Free-radical damage to the protein in connective tissue can cause stiffness in the body.

The "oxidative stress" inflicted by free radicals on tissues is similar to the oxidation of metal that leads to rusting. Or the oxidation of a fat, such as butter, that turns it rancid.

Besides the natural processes inside the body that generate damaging oxidative stress, free radical activity can also be increased and raised to dangerous overload level by lifestyle and environmental factors. They include alcohol; air pollution; chemical contaminants; chemotherapy; certain pharmaceutical drugs; excess exposure to sunlight; pesticides; physical and emotional stress; processed, smoked, or barbecued foods; and smoking.

The body fights back with antioxidants, compounds that counteract free radicals. Your cells make antioxidants, and you can also get antioxidants from food, notably fruits and vegetables, and supplements. It's when free radicals are not contained at a tolerable level by antioxidants that they set off their destructive blitz of oxidation.

Antioxidant

A molecule that converts free radicals into harmless chemicals like oxygen and water. Antioxidants are said to "quench" or "scavenge" free radicals, and thus neutralize them.

Many years ago, Denham Harman, M.D., Ph.D., theorized that vitamins such as E and C could counteract free radical activity in the body and thereby slow the aging process because these nutrients were found to have antioxidant properties. Harman's subsequent research demonstrated for the first time that feeding a variety of antioxidants to mammals could extend their lifespans.

There is now a massive volume of scientific evidence demonstrating that people who eat a diet high in antioxidants and who take antioxidant supplements will live longer, healthier lives.

"You can halt and even reverse many of the age-related problems that can arise (and make life so miserable) when our bodies suffer from an over-abundance of free radicals and a deficit of antioxidants," says Lester Packer, Ph.D., of the University of California at Berkeley, and a renowned authority on antioxidants.

Super Antioxidants

Hundreds of antioxidants have been identified, and until recently, these compounds were thought to work independently of one another. However, at Packer's world-famous laboratory, scientists have discovered that a few of them have a unique and dynamic interplay that greatly strengthens their individual effectiveness.

The members of this select super group are CoQ_{10}, glutathione, lipoic acid, and vitamins C and E. Packer calls them *network antioxidants*.

"Network antioxidants have special powers that set them apart from other antioxidants," says Packer in his book *The Antioxidant Miracle* (John Wiley & Sons, 1999). "They are particularly effective in slowing down the aging process and boosting the body's ability to fight disease. The antioxidant network is a shield that protects the body against the forces that age us before our time and rob years from our lives."

Vitamins C and E must be obtained in food. They are not produced by the body. However, to obtain an optimum antioxidant level of these vitamins through food is virtually impossible. And while we make our own CoQ_{10}, glutathione, and lipoic acid, the levels decrease as we age.

"That is why we need to supplement all of them," says Packer. "More than 70 percent of Americans will die prematurely from diseases caused by, or compounded by deficiencies of the antioxidant network," he contends.

Why CoQ_{10} Is So Special

Across the ocean from Packer's antioxidant laboratory in California, a group of Australian scientists at the Heart Research Institute in Sydney have brought to light some of the qualities of CoQ_{10} that make it so special.

Under the direction of Roland Stocker, Ph.D., they made the fascinating discovery that vitamin E itself can become a highly energized and reactive compound when it "scavenges" free radicals.

"Vitamin E can became a 'hot coal,' potentially damaging other molecules, unless it is brought back to a stable condition by a further partner in a chain which eventually terminates the process," says Stocker. Such partners are CoQ_{10} and vitamin C.

Researchers at the Australian institute have also demonstrated that CoQ_{10} is a primary antioxidant protector of low-density lipoproteins (known as LDL, or so-called harmful cholesterol). In one 1992 study on healthy young adults, they found that CoQ_{10} generated a "remarkable resistance" of LDL to oxidative damage. Too much oxidized LDL is damaging to the body because it leads to the formation of artery-narrowing plaque, a contributing condition for heart attacks and strokes.

A later study, conducted in Italy and published in the *Proceedings of the National Academy of Sciences USA*, suggested that CoQ_{10} may, in fact, be far more effective than any other antioxidant in blocking LDL oxidation.

The Super Mitochondria Protector

Over the years, many laboratory and clinical studies have yielded mounting evidence that supplemental CoQ_{10} offers a broad spectrum of protection against free radical activity. Research has shown it can protect, not just the arteries, but the brain, liver, muscles, nerves, and other systems in the body.

Much of this ability has to do with CoQ_{10}'s most critical antioxidant performance: inside the mitochondrial membranes where bioenergetics takes place.

Years ago, as Denham Harman evolved his free radical theory of aging, he introduced the idea that free radicals generated in the mitochondria "have the power to kill us." For that reason, he emphasized the importance of getting antioxidants into the mitochondria.

Today, a great deal of research has confirmed this concept. In fact, mitochondrial disease has become a booming segment of medical research and is being seen as a major cause of many degenerative conditions.

Along with this increased scientific interest has emerged a parallel interest in CoQ_{10} research because of its central contributions to mitochondrial "business." In the next chapter, we will see yet another contribution.

CHAPTER 4

THE GREAT ANTIAGING "SECRET"

So far we've seen that you need CoQ_{10} to keep you energized. Just like the spark in the engine of a car. We've also seen that it's a super antioxidant snuffing out damaging free radicals throughout the body and notably the torrent unleashed by energy production in trillions of cells.

So, CoQ_{10} sparks your engine, and prevents it from oxidizing and "rusting." Using the automotive analogy one more time, now we'll see how CoQ_{10} also puts the brakes on the aging process.

Turning Around Ailing, Aging Patients

Peter Langsjoen, M.D., has been prescribing CoQ_{10} to patients since the mid-1980s. "A large number of my patients are elderly and are doing great just on CoQ_{10} alone," he says. "You can't believe how active, healthy, and happy they are on virtually no medicine.

"When I see new patients in their 80s, coming in on walkers, I try to simplify their drugs if they are on a bunch of things, and I put them on CoQ_{10}. These are individuals who have been declining gradually and feeling poorly for a very long time. Typically, when I see them back again in six or eight weeks,

Aging
A complex biological process over time marked by a progressive decline in the performance of individual tissues and organs, and leading to age-associated disease and senility.

they are different people. They can't believe how much better they feel, and how fast it has happened. It makes the practice of medicine very gratifying."

Half a world away from Texas, down under in Australia, a distinguished molecular biologist named Anthony W. Linnane, Ph.D., has repeatedly shown in scientific studies how CoQ_{10} can turn aging and ailing patients like this around so dramatically.

Linnane is director of the Center for Molecular Biology and Medicine in Melbourne, a non-profit medical research institution. Interestingly, he started his career studying mitochondria in the very same University of Wisconsin laboratory where Fred Crane discovered CoQ_{10} . . . and at around the same time.

In 1989, Linnane published a theory in the prestigious medical journal *Lancet* that elaborated on Denham Harman's earlier proposal that the aging process actually begins in the mitochondria. He called his theory, "the universality of bioenergetic disease."

If you happened to skip over the last two chapters, I suggest you go back and read about the mitochondria, and the process of bioenergetics and free radical mayhem that goes on there. The information is key to understanding how CoQ_{10} works and also provides a background for what follows here.

The DNA Connection

The nucleus of cells, as we also know, contain the DNA that gives us our genetic heritage. For years, most scientists thought this was where aging originated.

Nuclear DNA can defend itself pretty well against free radical damage. It has good repair mechanisms. Mitochondria also have a genetic system of their own. This system, in concert with nuclear DNA, is required to maintain functional mitochondria. But unlike nuclear DNA, the genetic material inside mitochondria is much less efficient in repelling the flood of free radicals generated by the energy process.

Moreover, random mutations in mitochondrial

DNA occur throughout a life of ongoing replication and increase with advancing age.

Where Aging Really Takes Place

Free-radical damage increases with age as new generations of defective mitochondria replicate. Less and less energy is produced as a result. "Progressive depletion of energy production . . . is associated with the gradual decline of the physiological and biochemical performance of organs, significantly contributing to the aging process and ultimately to death," says Linnane.

In his research, the Australian molecular scientist repeatedly observed mutated mitochondria in yeast organisms, and then in the cells of laboratory animals and humans. "If you take a culture of yeast and grow them overnight, the next morning you have some mutants among them," he says. "Most of the cells will be normal, but a percentage won't be normal.

Mitochondrial Mutations: An Important Aspect of Aging

"We are basically no different. We are just an aggregation of cells, like a bacteria or yeast culture, but we are specialized, a collection of liver cells, muscle cells, or brain cells, but fundamentally the processes are the same.

"As our cells divide, more mutation occurs. The mutations add up over time. Energy degrades. We progressively lose power. And not only power, like in muscle power, but our metabolism begins to degrade as well. So, one important feature of aging, in my concept, is that we bioenergetically degrade because of mitochondrial mutation."

In other words, Linnane believes that the progressive accumulation of ongoing mitochondrial DNA mutation with age leads to a decline in cellular/ tissue bioenergy which, in turn, contributes to pathology. And in particular, he has in mind degenerative diseases of the blood vessels, brain, heart, and muscles.

CoQ$_{10}$ to the Rescue

Researchers, including Linnane, have experimented with CoQ$_{10}$ supplementation and find it inhibits the degradation and generates a partial re-energization of aging cells. This can help minimize the effects of aging and age-related diseases, they believe.

In one experiment with a long-lived breed of laboratory mice, researchers at UCLA found that the rodents supplemented with CoQ$_{10}$ after birth demonstrated a far greater level of activity as older animals than a non-supplemented group, and lived, on average, 20 percent longer.

Linnane has worked with Franklin Rosenfeldt, M.D., an Australian cardiology researcher, in both animal and human studies that have dramatically demonstrated the CoQ$_{10}$ relationship to mitochondrial stress, decline, and aging.

In one study, they experimented with specimens of heart tissue taken from patients of different ages who had been through heart surgery. In the laboratory, the specimens were exposed to oxygen deprivation and simulated ischemia, that is, interruption of blood flow. Later, the specimens were examined to determine how well they recovered from the ordeal.

It is well recognized that younger patients recovery faster from a heart attack or cardiac surgery than elderly patients, so it came as no surprise that the tissues taken from older patients demonstrated inferior recovery. In addition, the researchers found a strong connection between the integrity of the mitochondrial DNA in the tissue and the recovery rate.

Differences between Old and Young Tissue Eliminated

In a subsequent study, they then exposed heart tissue to CoQ$_{10}$ and subjected the specimens to the stress of simulated ischemia. Now, they reported, the difference in recovery between the tissue of older and younger patients was "abolished."

In yet another dramatic demonstration of CoQ_{10} power, they supplemented one group of old rats for six weeks and then put the animals through simulated aerobic exercise. Afterward, they compared the CoQ_{10} rodents to non-supplemented rats, both older and younger, who also went through the exercise trial.

The researchers found that the supplemented older rats performed and recovered just as well as the young rats. Moreover, these older rats on CoQ_{10} exhibited four times as much work capacity as the non-supplemented older rats. "We were astounded by the results," says Linnane.

In continuing studies, Linnane, Rosenfeldt, and their Australian colleagues have worked with human patients and further demonstrated the remarkable ability of CoQ_{10} to rekindle mitochondrial firepower and recovery. You will read more about their amazing findings in the next chapter.

CoQ_{10} and Antiaging Genes

In Anthony Linnane's latest research, he has opened an entirely new chapter on CoQ_{10}'s antiaging potential. Not only does CoQ_{10} function as an energizer and antioxidant in the mitochondria, but Linnane now believes it also activates the genes in the nuclear DNA to combat disease and essentially "turn back the clock" in cells.

Genes
A unit of DNA, the biochemical information database carrying the complete instructions for making all the proteins in a cell. Each gene contains specific instructions to make a particular protein.

CoQ_{10} does this by sending a chemical messenger to the nucleus. The process is far too complicated to explain here, but the messenger, it turns out, is actually a free radical called a peroxide that switches on certain strategic genes. The result is to fortify cellular systems in places where they have degraded, for instance, through the aging process. Thus, CoQ_{10} acts as a general regulator of cell metabolism to help maintain vital cellular functions.

"A powerful reaction sweeps across the whole of cellular metabolism, and weakened cells suddenly develop renewed strength and vitality," says Linnane. He believes this is how CoQ_{10} additionally benefits people suffering from a wide variety of conditions, from cancer to chronic fatigue and heart disease.

"People have never been able to understand how CoQ_{10} can do so many things that are reported in the anecdotal medical literature," he says. "This particular action could be the missing component that explains CoQ_{10}'s impact on so many healing fronts."

Making Muscles Younger

His latest study, published in the journal *Free-Radical Research* in 2002, offers a first-ever glimpse into how CoQ_{10} can regulate genes. The study made use of excised thigh-muscle tissue routinely removed from patients during hip replacement surgery. Such tissue is normally discarded.

But Linnane and his colleagues had a better use for the discards. First, they selected a group of older patients scheduled for this type of surgery at a Melbourne hospital. The patients were then randomly assigned to take either 300 mg of CoQ_{10} or an inert pill called a placebo. They were to follow this routine daily for the month before surgery.

After each surgery, the researchers collected the removed muscle tissue and put the specimens through a comprehensive series of analyses. They then compared the tissue taken from supplemented and non-supplement patients.

"What we found was very exciting," says Linnane. "We found that CoQ_{10} could change gene expression, that is, modulate gene expression in a significant way."

Specifically, they discovered that, after just one month, the muscle tissue taken from aging patients who were supplemented with CoQ_{10} was beginning to change toward a more youthful profile.

The First-Ever Physiological Change from CoQ_{10} Supplementation

In general, the quadriceps and other muscles are made up of different fiber types, like ropes, that slide across each other. The types are called slow- and fast-twitch fibers. As we age, we lose muscle tissue, but the fast type, associated with explosive strength, is progressively lost at a faster rate than slow-twitch muscles, which are associated with endurance.

"As we looked at the fibers in these specimens we could clearly see they were different from the fiber profile of a young person," says Linnane. "But when we compared the fibers of the elderly patients who were supplemented and those who were not, we found that the supplementation produced a dramatic change toward a younger profile.

"Mind you, the supplemented tissue didn't go back to a state you could say was a young profile, and we didn't make elderly people young again, but the CoQ_{10} generated degrees of change in that direction," he adds. "Along with that, the supplemented people told us they began to feel better, stronger, and more energized."

The study, Linnane says, is the first demonstration of an actual physiological change from CoQ_{10} supplementation.

"Huge" Antiaging Potential

"In order to do that, you would have to switch on a number of genes," Linnane explains. "You can't change muscle fiber otherwise. Hundreds of genes are required to make a muscle fiber. So, we found that CoQ_{10} modulated the genes relevant to muscle biochemistry and function, switching them back toward the re-creation of a somewhat younger profile.

This is a striking result that clearly warrants more research and more funding."

Linnane says that such changes wouldn't continue indefinitely and would likely reach a plateau. Still, he was delighted that a change of this nature was seen in only one month.

"CoQ_{10} makes cells stronger, more energized, and more competent to combat a wide range of diseases, and perhaps even prevent degenerative diseases that develop over long periods of time," he says.

"The research suggests that CoQ_{10} may dynamically support and strengthen the remaining physiological assets in an aging person. It can't put back what's gone, but hopefully it may slow the whole process. We need further research to clarify this.

"The key to all these marvelous functions of CoQ_{10} is that the substance be present in enough quantity. We know that as the body ages, there is less and less of it, so that's where supplementation comes in."

When asked about the importance of CoQ_{10} as an antiaging factor, Linnane answers unequivocally: "It has a huge potential. Supplementation is clearly indicated to improve the quality of life of older people and to provide protection against many age-related conditions."

From a clinical standpoint, doctors who use CoQ_{10} in their practice, believe strongly that CoQ_{10} indeed protects and rejuvenates.

"I see people with heart conditions and many other additional problems and they tell me that they have their life back, that they have renewed spark and energy," says Connecticut cardiologist Stephen Sinatra. "Their quality of life as a result of taking CoQ_{10}, whether they have heart disease or not, or whether they have chronic fatigue, or are just elderly and moving slower, will improve with CoQ_{10}."

(CHAPTER 5)

KEEPING YOUR HEART HEALTHY LONGER

It should not come as a surprise that the cells of the heart muscle are packed with mitochondria. In fact, they make up about a quarter of the volume in heart cells, more than anywhere else in the body.

That's obviously Nature's way of generating the power necessary to drive the heart's non-stop pumping action over a lifetime. Talk about a work schedule!

Your heart pushes blood (with its essential cargo of oxygen and nutrients) through a 60,000-mile network of blood vessels to nourish your brain, your feet, and everything in between. Every day, the heart muscle expands and contracts about 100,000 times, recycling 2,000 gallons of blood through your body. In a year, it contracts 36 million times.

That takes a lot of energy, and, yes, a lot of CoQ_{10}.

Mitochondrial Mutations and the Aging Heart

In the last chapter, we have seen how mutations of mitochondrial DNA cause a loss of energy in cells, and contribute to weakness, disease, and aging. In one Japanese study published in the *Molecular and Cellular Biochemistry Journal,* researchers found an accelerated rate of mitochondrial mutation in aging human hearts, and markedly so over the age of eighty. They concluded that such mutations play an important role in ebbing cardiac function among older people, and particularly in heart failure.

Protection of mitochondrial DNA against oxidative damage is of "primary importance in preventing the age-associated decline in cardiac performance," they emphasized.

CoQ_{10}, we have learned in the last chapter, protects mitochondrial DNA and the energy process from damage. It's a major mover, shaker, and protector in the mitochondrial scheme of things, so it is rather sobering to realize that the heart's natural CoQ_{10} content at age eighty is less than half of what it is at twenty.

CoQ_{10} Deficiency Imperils the Heart

Starting in the 1970s, researchers discovered that people with heart diseases were usually deficient in CoQ_{10}. One study found deficiencies in three-fourths of 132 patients undergoing heart surgery.

The most extreme examples of deficiencies occur among patients with weak hearts, suffering from conditions such as cardiomyopathy or heart failure.

And it isn't just an age thing. A deficiency of CoQ_{10} imperils the performance of the heart at any age. Indeed, clinicians and researchers rescue ailing hearts (young and old alike) by overcoming a deficiency with CoQ_{10} supplementation. It works for teenagers with cardiomyopathy, baby boomers with blocked arteries, and octogenarians with failing hearts.

To date, more than thirty-five controlled clinical trials in Japan, Australia, Europe, and the United States have demonstrated significant benefit for angina, cardiomyopathy, congestive heart failure,

Cardiomyopathy
In cardiomyopathy, the heart muscle becomes inflamed, dilated or thicker and doesn't pump well. If the specific cause is not known, the condition is called primary cardiomyopathy. If the cause is related to a disease involving other organs or the heart, the condition is secondary cardiomyopathy.

coronary artery disease, heart attacks, and recovery from heart surgery. These studies involve thousands of patients. They indicate that CoQ_{10} supplementation has a significant role both for early and advanced cases of heart disease, which kills 2,000 Americans daily.

Research in recent years has also uncovered an alarming connection between the use of common heart drugs to lower cholesterol levels and a CoQ_{10} deficiency. Experts warn that the deficiency created by these drugs poses a dangerous risk to health and heart that is virtually unrecognized. We'll cover this important issue later in the chapter.

Using CoQ_{10} Is Like Watering a Dry Plant

Texas cardiologist Peter Langsjoen, M.D., has participated in CoQ_{10} studies since the early 1980s, when the initial clinical trials were conducted in this country. First with his cardiologist father Per, who passed away in 1993, and subsequently on his own in private practice, Langsjoen has logged more clinical usage of CoQ_{10} than any other American doctor.

"CoQ_{10} is the backbone of my cardiac practice," he says. "Frankly it's unthinkable for me to practice medicine without it. Based on my experience with some 10,000 patients, I can unequivocally say it's a powerful substance that can do a great deal of good for many people, and without any side effects.

"Using CoQ_{10} is like watering a dry plant," he adds. "It's that remarkable. And it's that powerful. The sicker the patient, the more striking the results.

"In 80 percent of my patients, I see a clinical improvement in four weeks, with maximum improvement in six to twelve months, when they reach a plateau and have no further cardiovascular benefits. As their heart function improves, we have to decrease other medicines."

Langsjoen says that CoQ_{10}'s "most powerful therapeutic application is for any impairment in heart muscle function because the heart uses such a huge amount of energy. That's where you see the very dramatic lifesaving changes.

"This includes ischemic (lack of oxygen) conditions, such as coronary artery disease, because the CoQ_{10} energizes the viable cells left in the heart muscle.

"We really see across-the-board benefits. CoQ_{10} can help a big part of the population. This is a huge heart supplement."

A Boon for Heart Failure and Cardiomyopathy Patients

When the heart can't pump enough blood to the body the condition is called congestive heart failure, or simply heart failure. This life-threatening situation can result from narrowed arteries, a past heart attack that causes scarring and diminished efficiency of the heart muscle, high blood pressure, a congenital heart defect (present at birth), or cardiomyopathy.

Swelling (edema) often results, typically in the legs and ankles. Fluid can build up in the lungs and interfere with breathing, causing shortness of breath. The condition also impairs the kidneys' ability to dispose of sodium and water, leading to increased edema.

Drugs, including diuretics, are the standard treatment. When that fails, a patient may become a candidate for a heart transplant.

In the early 1980s, Karl Folkers, the biochemist who first identified the chemical structure of CoQ_{10}, collaborated with Per Langsjoen, who at the time was associated with The Scott and White Clinic in Temple, Texas. Together, they conducted the first well-controlled medical study of CoQ_{10} in the treatment of cardiomyopathy.

The effect of CoQ_{10} supplementation on the nineteen patients in the study was astounding. All were expected to die from heart failure, but they rebounded with an "extraordinary clinical improvement," the researchers declared. Hearts decreased in size, became more efficient, and pumped more blood. Heart Failure, including all forms of cardiomyopathy, seem to respond to CoQ_{10}, Per Langsjoen observed.

"CoQ_{10} is not specific to any type of heart failure," he added. "All forms of cardiomyopathy seem to respond to CoQ_{10}, including idiopathic (unknown cause), dilated (enlarged heart) or ischemic (reduced blood flow) cardiomyopathy."

Improved Quality of Life and Long-Term Survival

Subsequent research has confirmed the foregoing conclusion. Results include significantly improved quality of life and long-term survival from therapeutic supplementation.

One study analyzed the data compiled in eight previous controlled studies and found that patients supplemented with CoQ_{10} had better scores in five key measurements of heart performance than the vast majority of non-supplemented patients. Moreover, CoQ_{10} was found to be remarkably safe.

In 1994, the largest study with CoQ_{10} and heart-failure patients was reported in the journal *Molecular Aspects of Medicine*. In this trial, researchers at different Italian medical centers gave more than 2,500 patients CoQ_{10} in the amount of 50 to 150 mg daily for three months. The majority took 100 mg.

Improved quality of life was reported by 78 percent of the patients. Fifty-four percent attained significant improvement in at least three clinical signs that included general fluid retention, pulmonary fluid retention, heart palpitations, liver enlargement, and shortness of breath.

Such positive outcomes, along with many documented clinical reports, prompted Folkers to issue a strong appeal for the use of CoQ_{10} among individuals considering heart transplants.

Writing in the journal *Biochemical and Biophysical Research Communications*, Folkers argued that research has clearly "established the efficacy and safety of CoQ_{10} to treat patients in heart failure. In the United States, about 20,000 patients under sixty-five years are eligible for transplants, but donors number less than 1/10th of those eligible, and there are many more such patients over sixty-five, both eligible and ineligible."

CoQ_{10} Deficiency: The Dominant Cause of Heart Failure?

In his report, Folkers, along with both Per and Peter Langsjoen, described the results of eleven transplant candidates treated with CoQ_{10}. "After CoQ_{10}, all improved," they said. "Some patients required no conventional drugs and had no limitation in lifestyle."

One of the case histories they reported was a sixty-four-year-old African-American male with a failing heart and inoperable coronary disease. After six months, he had improved to the point where there was "no limitation whatsoever on his activities."

Many such dramatically positive cases like this, combined with the absence of side effects, "justify treating patients in failure . . . with CoQ_{10}," the researchers said.

Heart failure has been strongly correlated with low blood and tissue levels of CoQ_{10}. The more severe the disease, the greater the CoQ_{10} deficiency. This evidence led Folkers to theorize that the actual molecular cause of cardiac failure may be a "dominant deficiency" of CoQ_{10}.

"Even if you treat a patient with a conventional drug, the CoQ_{10} deficiency still remains," he said. "There is no cardiovascular drug that can do for the human body what CoQ_{10} can do."

The Most Dramatic Results

Peter Langsjoen agrees: "Among really complicated, critically ill cardiac patients who have been through one, two, or maybe three bypass procedures, you know that nothing really works. They are on a handful of drugs. But they feel terrible all the time.

"In this group we find the most dramatic results. These are the people who are the most severely deficient. The CoQ_{10} deficiency may well indeed be a primary causal factor in some types of heart muscle dysfunction while in others it may be a secondary phenomenon.

"No matter which, the deficiency appears to be a major treatable element in the otherwise relentless decline of heart failure."

Can Supplementation Minimize the Urgency for Heart Transplants?

It's astounding to think that a simple nutritional supplement can restore to normal a patient who is in line for a heart transplant. Yet it can, for young and old patients alike.

Langsjoen recalls the case several years ago of a New Jersey man who called on behalf of his ailing teenage son. The youngster had dilated cardiomyopathy, had been placed on medication, and had been told he would require a heart transplant within a year or so. His ejection fraction was 8 percent.

Ejection Fraction
The amount of blood your heart squeezes out into the bloodstream with each beat. Generally speaking, an ejection fraction reading of 50 percent or more is regarded as healthy.

"The father had done his homework and knew about CoQ_{10}," Langsjoen says. "He contacted me to find out if it could help his son. We sent him reprints of CoQ_{10} studies on this type of condition. The father went ahead, with the agreement of his son's physician, and had the boy take 300 mg daily.

"Several months later, I heard again from the father. He was quite excited. His son's ejection fraction had gone to 24 percent. The last I heard, it was 34 percent, and the boy was beginning to do light jogging. This is obviously a striking change."

In this particular case, the youngster had just been diagnosed. Can CoQ_{10} help with very advanced disease?

"When you catch people early, the heart muscle hasn't yet deteriorated with fibrous tissue and scarring," says Langsjoen. "If someone has had a large, weak heart for years, it is unusual to get those hearts back to normal. You gradually lose heart muscle cells and you don't regrow them. A scarred heart is a tough situation.

"If the cells are weak, but alive, you then have the potential to improve them. You can gradually improve heart function for a year or two. That means decreasing heart size and increasing ejection fraction. Normally, after a year there is a leveling off."

And do patients have to continue the CoQ_{10} once they have improved?

"They should not stop taking it," Langsjoen answers. "I have had patients who were doing well and decided they didn't need the supplement anymore. Usually within a month's time there is measurable decline. This has been the observation of other experts as well. I haven't seen them worse than when they started, but subjectively there is a decline and if you look at their CoQ_{10} blood levels, there is a matching drop as well."

Coronary Artery Disease

Heart attacks usually result from coronary artery disease, also known as coronary or ischemic (*is-kem-ik*) heart disease. This condition is the single largest killer of American men and women, causing more than 450,000 deaths a year.

A heart attack occurs when the blood supply to part of the heart muscle is severely reduced or blocked off. This happens when one or more of the four coronary arteries feeding blood to the heart become blocked. The common cause is a buildup of plaque on the arterial walls that is called atherosclerosis. These deposits narrow the arteries, gradually choke the flow of blood, and increase the prospect for clots to block circulation.

The consequences include sudden cardiac arrest (a heart attack) or angina, where tightness and pain are felt in the chest with physical activity, emotional disturbance, or even intense elation.

CoQ$_{10}$'s "Magic"

CoQ$_{10}$ won't unclog arteries, bring back to life dead heart muscle cells, or replace lifesaving heart drugs. But it does offer impressive benefits against atherosclerosis and coronary artery disease.

First of all, it re-energizes the heart cells, including those on the edge, cells in trouble that may either die or struggle to live on. "This is CoQ$_{10}$'s magic," says Connecticut cardiologist Stephen Sinatra, M.D. "It can rejuvenate those cells."

Let's say the heart muscle is getting poor blood flow, just enough to keep it pumping. With CoQ$_{10}$, it will function better with whatever limited flow it does have. A patient will definitely have less chest pain, in fact, quite a bit less. This is not because the arteries are being opened but rather because of better energy production in the functioning areas that are poorly supplied.

CoQ$_{10}$, as we've seen, is also a powerful antioxidant operating in the mitochondria where tremendous amounts of free radicals are produced.

In addition, CoQ$_{10}$ is present in the bloodstream, where it circulates with other antioxidants. As it circulates, it combines with vitamin E, another antioxidant, to help prevent lipid peroxidation. It also protects vitamin E itself from free radical destruction, a protective relationship that has been discovered only recently.

It turns out that CoQ$_{10}$ molecules in the bloodstream are actually transported by the LDL cholesterol. CoQ$_{10}$ protects the LDL from oxidation, something in the Wild West tradition of "riding shotgun" on the stagecoach.

Lipid Peroxidation

A scientific term for the damaging oxidation by free radicals on fatty substances inside the body. Such substances include the membranes of cells as well as LDL (low-density lipoprotein), the major cholesterol-bearing blood fat. When LDL cholesterol gets oxidized, it becomes a potentially harmful agent contributing to the development of artery-narrowing plaque.

Animal studies have demonstrated that CoQ_{10} supplementation significantly protects against dangerous arterial plaque, even when animals are fed diets designed to raise the level of cholesterol and other fats in their bodies.

Thus, CoQ_{10}'s antioxidant power benefits the heart itself and the blood vessels that supply it.

CoQ_{10} Reduces Angina Episodes

A number of controlled studies have shown that CoQ_{10} generates major improvements in exercise tolerance, and reduces the frequency of angina episodes and the need for medication as well.

Dosages in these studies range from 150 to 600 mg daily.

One study also showed that when CoQ_{10} is given to patients after a heart attack, it works quickly to lower the risk of complications and additional cardiac events. In this study, patients received 120 mg of CoQ_{10} within a few days of their heart attack.

After four weeks on CoQ_{10}, they had far less experience of angina, arrhythmias, and every other measure studied, when compared with a second group of heart attack patients who were not supplemented. The CoQ_{10} group had about half as many subsequent heart attacks during this time.

The Amazing Recovery of a Three-Bypass Patient

Texas cardiologist and CoQ_{10} expert Peter Langsjoen says that these types of patients do "so well" with

CoQ_{10}. As an example, he cited a female patient in her seventies who previously had three bypass surgeries. "Even after surgeries, she was having chest pain many times a day and was bedridden," he recalls. "Just to get up and get dressed she would have to take three or four nitroglycerine pills. She would get chest pain just sitting and watching TV.

"We started her on CoQ_{10}. Now, years later, she manages her own affairs and is quite active. She still has angina, but only from time to time. CoQ_{10} made a clear difference.

"This is somebody with extremely poor plumbing. Her arteries are a mess. Her grafts are a mess. There is nothing more to do surgically. You couldn't bypass her another time. I was amazed she even survived the third operation. Her heart is about as ischemic as you can get. We could never really improve someone in that shape without something like CoQ_{10}. She takes 120 mg twice a day along with other anti-angina medications."

Boosts Recovery after Cardiac Surgery

Supplementation with CoQ_{10} prior to heart surgery appears also to significantly help the recovery process.

"If a surgeon would like his heart patients to recover better and have a stronger heart muscle, CoQ_{10} supplementation should be a real option to use," says Franklin Rosenfeldt, M.D., of the Alfred Hospital Cardiac Surgical Research Unit in Melbourne.

Rosenfeldt has conducted multiple studies proving CoQ_{10} improves surgical outcomes. In the latest

Coronary Artery Bypass Surgery
In this common cardiac procedure, the surgeon reroutes, or bypasses, blood around clogged coronary arteries to improve the supply of blood and oxygen to the heart. A blood vessel is taken from another part of the body and grafted above and below the blocked part of the affected coronary artery.

study, 122 patients scheduled for elective coronary artery bypass graft (CABG) surgery were randomly selected to take either CoQ_{10} or an inert placebo pill for one week before their operation. The amount of CoQ_{10} used in the study was 300 mg a day.

After the surgery, the researchers found that CoQ_{10} generated impressive results, including improved mitochondrial energy production, better heart muscle contraction, less heart muscle damage, and less recovery time in the hospital.

Major Implications for Life and Cost-Saving

"This is very promising and very effective in many cases," says Rosenfeldt, who reported his findings at a scientific conference of the American Heart Association in 2001.

Langsjoen emphatically agrees. "This is a great result," he points out, "obtained after just seven days. From my own experience of using CoQ_{10} for several months or so before bypass surgery, I feel that the post-operative benefits can be even more substantial."

More than half-a-million bypass surgeries are performed in the United States each year. They involve increasingly older patients and an increasing percentage of repeat operations. As a result, the injury, death and cost burden have risen substantially.

A number of studies have shown that pretreatment with CoQ_{10} improves the postoperative status of patients not just after bypass surgery, but also after heart valve replacement as well. Hopefully, cardiologists will recognize the value that CoQ_{10} can contribute to surgical outcomes and heart health in general. Up to now, however, they haven't paid much attention.

The Danger of Cholesterol-Lowering Drugs

These days the advertisements for cholesterol-lowering drugs are totally in your face. They pop up everywhere. In magazines, newspapers, and TV. And the message coming out of the pharmaceutical industry is that even healthy people should take these drugs, known technically as statins. They are, in fact, being touted as the "new aspirin."

Statins
These cholesterol-lowering drugs were introduced in 1987 and have become blockbuster drugs with total annual sales now over $14 billion. Leading products include Pfizer's Lipitor, Merck's Zocor, and Bristol-Myers Squibb's Pravachol.

Beyond the smoke of marketing hype, a threatening fire smolders. In 2001, major headlines and news reports warned users of these drugs about the potential for deadly muscle damage. One leading statin brand, *Baycol,* was voluntarily pulled off the market by its manufacturer in the summer of 2001 after thirty-one deaths were linked to its usage. Public Citizen, a well-known consumer advocacy group, also petitioned the U.S. Food and Drug Administration (FDA) to require manufacturers to warn patients to quit the pills at the first sign of muscle pain or weakness.

What the Media Hasn't Reported
What has not been brought to public attention is that these drugs also interfere with the body's production of CoQ_{10}. They block the same enzyme system (known as HMG-CoA) that produces both cholesterol *and* CoQ_{10}.

"It is almost criminal, in my opinion, not to supplement a person who is taking statin drugs," says cardiologist Stephen Sinatra. "The drugs are creating CoQ_{10} deficiencies. The *Baycol* problem is just the tip of the iceberg. Animal studies show that statins can lead to cancer."

In his medical practice, Sinatra will only prescribe

a statin drug to a very sick cardiac patient who cannot otherwise reduce his or her cholesterol by natural means.

An Impending Medical Disaster?

"But I always prescribe CoQ_{10} along with it," Sinatra adds. "Any person taking a statin *must* take CoQ_{10}. The problem is that these drugs are big business and promoted to healthy people all over the place, and doctors aren't telling their patients about the CoQ_{10} connection. A lot of people are taking the drugs preventively but could be literally awakening a tiger inside the body that could come alive later on in life."

Says cardiologist Peter Langsjoen: "This could be the biggest impending medical disaster ever."

Experts commonly see the signs of CoQ_{10} deficiency in new patients who have been taking statin drugs for a year or more.

Warning Signs Are Deceiving

Typical signs include aches and pains, fatigue, malaise, sore muscles, weakness, difficulty getting in and out of a car, the feeling of a low-grade flu, and shorter breath with exertion. There could be mental changes as well.

The signs are deceiving and people may not link them to the cholesterol drug. With statins, the experts say, you don't have any immediate side effects. You get the immediate gratification that cholesterol is coming down, but over time you start feeling less well and just don't attribute it to something you started a year or two before.

Moreover, adds Langsjoen, echocardiograph imaging of the heart will show an abnormality of

Echocardiography
Ultrasound imaging technology used by cardiologists to help assess heart function, heart wall thickness, and the severity of disorders.

the heart muscle function in these people, specifically a stiffening of the heart muscle.

"This is the very first thing you see with CoQ_{10} depletion," he says. "It is very common in people on statins for any length of time. It is reversible, and goes back to normal if you stop the drug."

FDA Informed about the Danger

Mounting studies proving that statin drugs seriously deplete CoQ_{10} prompted The International Coenzyme Q_{10} Association to bring the issue to the attention of the FDA in September of 2001.

In a letter to the FDA signed by fourteen scientists and clinicians in seven countries, the group pointed out that muscle destruction and fatigue linked to the drugs may in fact be a direct result of depletion. The scientists also noted that although statin therapy has benefits, its long-term benefits against heart disease may be "blunted" due to the depletion of CoQ_{10}.

Finally, the association urged the FDA to study "whether the clinical use of statins can be made safer and possibly more effective by the addition of CoQ_{10}. We should make every effort to investigate the reasons for, and to prevent further developments of what have already been serious medical consequences."

CHAPTER 6

IF IT'S SO GOOD, WHY AREN'T CARDIOLOGISTS USING IT?

In October of 1996, Connecticut cardiologist Stephen Sinatra received an urgent call from a man who pleaded with him to take his mother in transfer from another hospital. The woman was seventy-nine-years-old at the time and had been admitted to a community hospital with heart failure complicated by pneumonia.

The son said she had been on a ventilator for several weeks, was getting powerful steroids and high concentrations of oxygen, but was still failing. She went into kidney failure and her doctors said there was nothing more to do.

The son, who placed the S-O-S call to Sinatra, was a biochemist and knowledgeable about CoQ_{10}. He had asked the doctors at the hospital to place his mother on CoQ_{10}. They refused. CoQ_{10} was not on their list of approved formulas.

The son brought in stacks of medical literature showing how CoQ_{10} could help patients with heart failure. The doctors would not review the information. Instead, they asked the family to end life support. The family refused.

The son went to the hospital administrators. When he insisted on the CoQ_{10}, they told him he was "interfering." The situation turned ugly, and lawyers became involved.

A Happy Ending

The story, however, had a happy ending. Sinatra told the son that if his mother could be transferred to a hospital where he could attend to her, he would see to it that she received CoQ_{10}. CoQ_{10} was approved for use at the Connecticut hospital Manchester Memorial.

Still, he warned, the transfer was risky in her weakened state. She would have to be transported in an ambulance for the forty-or-so-minute journey and be "bag-breathed" the whole way. This meant that a skilled medical technician would have to "breathe" her mechanically by hand the entire time.

The son was quick to respond. "At least with you she will have a fighting chance because, where she is, she's certainly going to die," he said.

The transfer was carried out. The elderly woman arrived, semi-comatose, and respiratory-dependent. She was placed on conventional pulmonary care similar to that received at the previous hospital.

Conventional Treatment *Plus* Supplements

The only change in her therapy was nutritional: 450 mg of CoQ_{10} daily, given through a feeding tube, along with a multivitamin/mineral preparation, and one gram of magnesium, intravenously administered.

"Although I had some hope for her, the other critical care doctors were extremely skeptical of using CoQ_{10} in this life-threatening case," Sinatra says.

On the third day, she started to "wake up." After ten days, she was weaned off the ventilator. At two weeks, she was discharged to an extended care facility, sitting up in a wheelchair with only supplemental oxygen.

Sinatra has seen Louise on a number of occasions since then. She is now eighty-three and enjoying a good quality of life. She requires routine medical therapy but also takes 500 mg of CoQ_{10} daily.

In Sinatra's words, what happened was "truly a medical resurrection" and represents the great life-saving potential of CoQ_{10}.

But the story is not unusual, he says: "I have personally treated and heard of many cases of people seemingly 'left for dead' who have been similarly res-urrected by this remarkable compound called CoQ_{10}."

Only a Small Minority of Cardiologists Use CoQ_{10}

In Japan, CoQ_{10} is the fifth most commonly pre-scribed heart "drug." Japanese cardiologists know its value. Up until recently it was available only through prescription there, but as of 2001 it can be bought as an over-the-counter supplement just as in the United States. Here, however, most cardiologists ignore CoQ_{10}.

"Probably less than 1 percent of cardiologists know it and use it," guesses Sinatra. "The rest are simply missing a great therapeutic tool."

How can this be, given the proven success of CoQ_{10} in scientific studies, and the excitement and gratification it generates among patients?

Why They Are Missing the Boat

One major reason is that CoQ_{10} is "only" a nutrition-al supplement and not a patented drug. In Western medicine, the pharmaceutical companies dominate medical practice. They research and develop drugs, patent them, and market them to practitioners, who prescribe them to patients.

Health professionals, and particularly specialists, tend to treat patients according to the accepted pro-tocols of their specialty. The protocols emphasize medical technology and pharmaceutical drugs, not nutritional supplements.

The official position of the American Heart Asso-ciation is that "the safety and effectiveness of CoQ_{10} need to be further evaluated. This requires conduct-ing well-designed clinical trials involving large num-bers of patients over a long time. Until that happens, the American Heart Association cannot recommend taking coenzyme Q_{10} regularly."

Dozens of heart-related studies from around the

world overwhelmingly show that CoQ_{10} is very safe and effective. For very sick people, however, it needs to be used in high enough doses to achieve healing blood levels. But obviously, in the current medical environment, nutritional supplements, no matter how vital or how essential, typically get short shrift. They are ignored or relegated to minor importance even though medical drugs often cause nutrient deficiencies in the body. CoQ_{10} is a prime "victim" of this approach.

Opposition from the Status Quo

Langsjoen adds this perspective: "While the pharmaceutical industry does a good job at physician and patient education on their new products, distributors of CoQ_{10} are not as effective at this. This education is very costly and can be done only with the reasonable expectation of patent-protected profit. CoQ_{10} is not patentable.

"Although this is not the first time that a fundamental and clinically important discovery has come about without the backing of a pharmaceutical company, it is the first such discovery to so radically alter how we as physicians must view disease. CoQ_{10} is not revolutionary in the fields of chemistry and biochemistry, but it is revolutionary in medical practice and as such there is inherent opposition from the status quo."

Until now, CoQ_{10} is best known outside of mainstream medicine—in alternative health circles. And a December 2000 report on ABC World News Tonight lamented that fact, citing the significant benefits to patients.

"Come on cardiologists!" chided ABC commentator Nicholas Regush. "Crack open the medical literature on coenzyme Q_{10}. Start reading up on how this powerful substance may be able to help patients with heart problems." Hopefully somebody was listening.

CHAPTER 7

HIGH BLOOD PRESSURE, STROKE, AND DIABETES

In addition to directly helping the heart, CoQ_{10} also benefits the cardiovascular system as a whole. That means the circulatory system as well. And in doing so, CoQ_{10} further adds to its value as both a natural preventive and therapeutic agent.

In this chapter we will discuss CoQ_{10}'s potential for three major conditions: high blood pressure (hypertension), stroke, and diabetes.

CoQ_{10} and High Blood Pressure

You are about to read some great news if you are among the approximately one in four adult Americans with high blood pressure. What you will learn is something your doctor likely doesn't know about . . . so show this to your physician.

First, the facts. Hypertension, or high blood pressure as it is popularly called, is not really a disease. It is a byproduct of other, often more serious, underlying problems.

High blood pressure means that the force of blood pressing against the walls of the arteries is too great. Fully one-third of the individuals with high blood pressure have no symptoms and don't even know they have it.

But symptoms or no symptoms, if not controlled, high blood pressure can lead to brain damage, heart attacks, heart failure, kidney disease, and stroke.

Causes Mostly Unknown and Treatments Largely Unsuccessful

In 90 percent of cases, the cause is not precisely

known and is referred to as essential hypertension. Among the causal factors are age, body weight, diet, heredity (high blood pressure is more common and severe among blacks than whites), kidney infection, and stress.

Only about 18 percent of those with high blood pressure are successfully treated. Moreover, many people fear the side effects of medication or improper prescribing by physicians.

What Determines High Blood Pressure

A person is considered to have high blood pressure when he or she has a systolic pressure of 140 mmHg or greater, and/or a diastolic pressure of 90 mmHg or greater, or is taking antihypertensive medication. *Systolic* means the pressure when the heart is beating. *Diastolic* means pressure between heartbeats. Eighty percent of people fall in the borderline-to-moderate range (120–180 over 90–114) and require no drug therapy at all. A normal blood pressure is 120 over 80.

Now that you have the facts, here is the exciting CoQ_{10} connection: As far back as 1976, researchers noted that CoQ_{10} could decrease blood pressure in patients with established hypertension. Over the years, the evidence has continued to grow, and now points to a possible CoQ_{10} deficiency as a *cause* of high blood pressure.

Based on years of using CoQ_{10} in their cardiology practices, Peter Langsjoen and his late father, Per, theorized that, with CoQ_{10} supplementation, improved heart functioning precedes lowered blood pressure.

Is Hypertension the Result of a CoQ_{10} Deficiency?

Here are the details: The heart muscle is packed with mitochondria and CoQ_{10}. In any disease that affects heart muscle function, whether it is coronary artery disease, diabetes, mitral valve disease, or the result of chemotherapy toxicity, the first change that occurs is a stiffening and thickening of the heart muscle. This phenomenon may very well be the result of a CoQ_{10} deficiency.

A deficiency is seen, for instance, as a result of the regular use of cholesterol-lowering drugs which deplete the body of CoQ_{10}. A depletion could also occur from polluted air, poor diet, and stress which cause shortages in important vitamins, such as B complex, necessary for the body to produce CoQ_{10}.

We know that CoQ_{10} production declines with age. And we also know that a stiffening of the heart muscle is considered a normal aspect of aging (a senile heart).

The Heart Has to Work Harder

The stiffening means the heart has to work harder in order to fill its chambers with blood and then pump it out again. In response, the body produces adrenaline, the stress hormone. It makes the heart rate higher and improves the filling and pumping action. However, on a continual basis, the increased adrenaline causes a general constriction of the blood vessels, which means that higher (more) blood pressure is required to push the blood through narrowed arteries.

> **Adrenaline**
>
> *Heightened secretion of this important adrenal hormone is often related to fear or anger, and results in an increased heart rate and the conversion of stored glycogen to glucose. This reaction, popularly known as the fight or flight response, sets up the body for intensified action.*

"We've always looked at essential hypertension as a disease that causes thickening of the heart muscle," says Langsjoen. "That's what the textbooks say. But the experts have never looked seriously at CoQ_{10}.

"From my clinical experience, it is the CoQ_{10} deficiency that is causing the stiffening of the heart muscle, which, in turn, causes the body to respond with adrenaline. The end result is hypertension."

The concept is revolutionary and certainly warrants major clinical trials with large numbers of patients.

Hundreds of Patients Normalized with CoQ_{10}

To date there have been about ten studies, most of them small. All have shown improvement in heart muscle function and gradual lowering of blood pressure.

At the Langsjoen clinic, hundreds of patients with mild to moderate hypertension have been normalized within three to six months on CoQ_{10} *alone*. The stiffness, the increased heart rate, and the blood pressure, "all go to normal," Langsjoen says.

The CoQ_{10} results are very powerful with younger people, aged twenty to forty, says Langsjoen. "In older people, there are usually more complications involved. Nevertheless, I would say that this concept applies to a fair amount of my patients with hypertension, and maybe even a majority."

In Connecticut, Stephen Sinatra has also achieved striking results. "Since using CoQ_{10} for more than ten years, I have been able to slowly reduce at least half their cardiac medications," he says.

As blood pressure gradually normalizes, patients are often able to start reducing the amount of medication they take. They report improvement in their quality of life and vigor. Obviously, CoQ_{10} is having an energizing effect, but improvement also occurs as a result of taking less medication.

In a 1994 report published in the journal *Molecular Aspects of Medicine,* Langsjoen described a clinical study with 109 symptomatic patients. These were advanced cases where the patients had had the condition an average of nine years.

Here, about 25 percent of those studied were eventually controlled on CoQ_{10} alone, 100 mg twice daily.

"People with severe hypertension are going to need drugs," he points out. "But you can always add some CoQ_{10} in their daily routine and often be able to reduce the drugs."

Think of CoQ_{10} as a Primary Therapeutic Resource

In an informal experiment in his clinic, Langsjoen took echocardiograms on sixteen older patients with elevated blood pressure who were not initially taking CoQ_{10}. The images all showed stiffening of the heart muscle, typical for their age. All of them normalized with CoQ_{10}. "If we can reverse the stiffening with CoQ_{10}, then hypertension may not be such an un-avoidable phenomenon in older people," he says.

Langsjoen suggests that patients with hypertension should bring CoQ_{10} to the attention of their physician. Because of its safety, effectiveness, and multiple benefits, he believes strongly that it should be considered prior to an escalating course of drugs.

"Consider CoQ_{10} in situations of mild or moderate hypertension, particularly when it is mild enough not to be symptomatic," he says. "You can expect to see a gradual improvement of 10 to 15 mmHg."

This promise of CoQ_{10} for hypertension takes on even greater importance in the light of new research findings showing that even slightly elevated blood pressure (in the range physicians call high normal) significantly raises the risk of heart disease. The findings, published in the *New England Journal of Medicine* in 2001, indicated the risk was 2.5 times higher than in individuals with lower normal readings, and increased with age.

"Even if blood pressure is quite high, symptoms are present, and medication is necessary, CoQ_{10} should be considered as a way of gradually decreasing the level of medicine," says Langsjoen.

"Keep in mind, however, that CoQ_{10} doesn't address all the multiple lifestyle factors that may have contributed to a person getting into the high-blood-pressure predicament to begin with. The stresses and other causal elements are still ongoing."

CoQ_{10} and Stroke

Stroke is the third leading killer disease, after coronary artery disease and cancer. It occurs when arteries to, or inside, the head become blocked, choking off circulation to a portion of the brain. A minor stroke may cause temporary loss of sensory or organ function. But a major stroke can cause permanent paralysis, or even death.

Research into CoQ_{10} and stroke has been limited to animal studies. In these experiments, animals who were supplemented for a period prior to an induced stroke were much less injured than non-supplemented animals. A similar effect has been observed in humans but has not been formally studied.

Impressive Recoveries

Peter Langsjoen describes a better-than-expected recovery among his heart patients who were taking CoQ_{10} and happened to have a stroke.

"I have seen patients completely paralyzed on one side, and unable to speak, after a devastating stroke, and then after several months they get back to being pretty much normal," he says. "There might be some remaining clumsiness of the hand, or one leg not quite tracking as well, or some slight thing.

"I have seen impressive recoveries in dozens of patients, recoveries that have not only impressed me, but the physical therapy people as well."

Langsjoen says he usually increases the amount of CoQ_{10} after a stroke to about 180 mg twice daily.

"I don't have any experience with people who have not been on CoQ_{10} prior to a stroke, and then are put on it afterwards. At that point, it may be too late. Most of my patients take CoQ_{10}."

Along these same lines, John Ely, Ph.D., a research physics scientist at the University of Washington, reported the case of a remarkable recovery from a severe stroke by a sixty-nine-year-old female who had been taking 400 mg of CoQ_{10} for a month prior to having a stroke.

Ely, writing about the case in a 1998 issue of the *Journal of Orthomolecular Medicine*, said the patient recovered "almost completely" in two weeks despite the "vegetative prognosis foreseen by the very experienced stroke unit specialists" at the hospital.

CoQ_{10} and Diabetes

Remember Fred Crane? He's the retired researcher who first discovered CoQ_{10} in 1957. Many years later, Crane developed diabetes and required oral medication to control his blood sugar. But with time the medication wasn't working well. His blood sugar level began to rise again.

As Crane tells it, "I thought that maybe CoQ_{10} might help. I had been taking 30 mg a day, but then I stepped up to 180 mg. In a period of about six months, my insulin level normalized, and my blood sugar dropped down to about where it should be. I've been on this approach for seven years, taking my oral medication and the additional CoQ_{10}. And it's been working."

An Alarming Rise in Diabetes

The rising incidence of diabetes has health officials deeply concerned. Like Crane's case, the most common form of the disease develops slowly, usually among people over age forty-five.

The latest statistics from the Centers for Disease Control indicate that nearly 16 million Americans— 6 percent of the population—have diabetes, the highest level ever recorded. Moreover, the disease is developing at the staggering rate of 798,000 new cases a year.

Although diabetes is not a cardiovascular disease per se, it has a harmful impact on the cardiovascular system. It contributes to free radical activity and a systemic deterioration of blood vessels.

Diabetics Deficient in CoQ$_{10}$

Medical studies reveal a deficiency of CoQ$_{10}$ in diabetic patients. In one study, 120 mg per day of CoQ$_{10}$ was given to thirty-nine patients with diabetes, resulting in a reduction of blood-sugar levels by 20 to 30 percent.

At his Texas cardiology clinic, Peter Langsjoen has found that CoQ$_{10}$ has improved the blood-sugar-related problems of some of his heart patients who also have diabetes. He has not done a formal study, but during one stretch of time he carefully reviewed the progress of about 140 patients with adult-onset diabetes.

"About one-third of them were clearly doing better," he says. "By that I mean better blood-sugar control and a reduced need for medication. Among this group, patients went from insulin injections to pills, or from pills to control with diet alone." The diabetic symptoms of the other patients did not change significantly.

The CoQ$_{10}$ Connection Not Widely Known

The fact that CoQ$_{10}$ appears to help normalize blood sugar in a substantial number of cases is not well known. And clearly, much research is needed to clarify a potential role for CoQ$_{10}$.

"It appears to happen enough of the time that I inform patients they may need to substantially lower their level of insulin or oral medication," says Langsjoen.

The action of CoQ$_{10}$ is probably related to improving the bioenergetics and, as a result, the production of the so-called beta cells in the pancreas where insulin is made.

"With CoQ$_{10}$, you change the fundamental cellular chemistry of everything," he says. "So you see many improvements in the body. There are so many aspects of health that improve simply because you are energizing everything."

The Diabetes Supplement "Cocktail"

Connecticut cardiologist Stephen Sinatra uses CoQ$_{10}$ as part of an overall supplement approach to help patients with a family history of diabetes prevent the disease. He recommends a daily "cocktail" of the following:

- Alpha-lipoic acid, an antioxidant, 100–300 mg

- CoQ$_{10}$, 200–400 mg

- L-Carnitine, an amino acid, 1–2 grams

- Magnesium, 400 mg

- Vitamin E, 200–400 IU

"These nutrients will help prevent oxidative stress in the pancreas and also help control blood sugar," says Sinatra.

CHAPTER 8

KEEPING YOUR IMMUNE SYSTEM STRONG

Energizer, antioxidant, and mitochondria protector par excellence. That's CoQ_{10}. It shouldn't come as a surprise, then, that these remarkable properties of CoQ_{10} extend to the immune system, the body's wondrous defense mechanism.

Physicians say CoQ_{10} boosts resistance to disease. People get sick less often. They get fewer colds, flu, and respiratory infections. They are not as sickly. If they come down with a viral illness, it is much milder. CoQ_{10} may also represent a front-line natural agent against more serious disorders, such as AIDS and cancer.

Although the CoQ_{10} research in the area of immunology doesn't approach the volume of scientific work done in cellular bioenergetics and heart disease, the findings nevertheless suggest a good deal of promise for CoQ_{10}.

Fortified Antibodies and Immune Cells

Studies show, for instance, that CoQ_{10} can improve antibody levels. In one Italian study, a group of volunteers took either 90 or 180 mg of CoQ_{10} for two weeks prior to vaccination against the hepatitis-B virus. After vaccination, they continued taking the supplement for another ninety days.

Researchers then measured the antibody levels and compared them with another group of vaccinated volunteers which was not supplemented. Both dosages of CoQ_{10} effectively improved the antibody response and the higher supplementation level increased the response by up to 57 percent.

In another human study, involving eight chronically ill patients, supplementation with 60 mg of CoQ_{10} for up to three months significantly improved their levels of IgG, the body's most common antibody.

Other studies, done with laboratory animals, show that CoQ_{10} contributes to a greater killing ability for macrophages, immune cells that devour bac-

---

Antibodies

Specialized molecules made of proteins produced by immune system cells called lymphocytes. Antibodies circulate in the blood and lymph fluid where they bind to "foreign invaders" (bacteria, toxic substances, or viruses) that enter the body. The alien substances are inactivated, or identified for destruction by other immune cells. The body produces many different antibodies.

---

teria and viruses. These studies also show that an age-related decline in immune system function can be partially reversed with CoQ_{10} supplementation. Moreover, supplemented older animals become healthier and more energetic.

People and animals alike lose energy and resistance to illness as they age. Thus, older people should consider adding CoQ_{10} to their supplement arsenal of such illness-fighters as vitamins A and C.

CoQ_{10} and Cancer

Research on the CoQ_{10}-cancer connection is limited. There have been no controlled studies. But the medical observations made to date clearly call for the therapeutic benefits of CoQ_{10} to be vigorously studied.

Karl Folkers, Ph.D., one of the original scientists involved with CoQ_{10}, believed that CoQ_{10} should be aggressively explored for its cancer-protective effects. Since it is not a patented drug, however, funding for large-scale research has not materialized.

In Europe, studies have shown a low level of

CoQ_{10} in the blood and affected tissues of cancer patients.

Protective Effect for Breast Tissue

In one study, Turkish researchers noted the involvement of free radical damage (see Chapter 3) to cell membranes, mitochondria, and DNA in the cancer process. Increased free radical activity, they pointed out, could cause an excess consumption of CoQ_{10} by the body.

Analyzing cancerous breast tissue removed from twenty-one mastectomy patients, the researchers found a significantly decreased level of CoQ_{10}. They concluded that supplementation of CoQ_{10} "may induce a protective effect on breast tissue."

A small-scale 1994 Scandinavian study involving CoQ_{10} and "high-risk" breast cancer was reported in the journal *Biochemical and Biophysical Research Communication*. In that study, thirty-two patients were given an array of vitamins, antioxidants, fatty acids and 90 mg of CoQ_{10}, along with conventional cancer treatment.

An Amazing Tumor Regression

Six of the cases showed partial tumor regression. One of the six women, whose tumor had stabilized in size to 1.5 centimeters over a year, was then given an increased dosage of 390 mg of CoQ_{10}. According to the researchers, after one month the tumor was no longer palpable. In another month, mammography confirmed the absence of tumor.

One of the authors commented that in treating almost 7,000 cases of breast cancer over a thirty-five year practice, he had "never seen a spontaneous complete regression" of a breast tumor that size, and had "never seen a comparable regression on any conventional anti-tumor therapy."

Another woman in the study underwent non-radical surgery for a breast tumor, but her physicians determined the presence of residual cancer. She was then given 300 mg of CoQ_{10} daily. After three months, she was described as being in excellent clinical condition with no evidence of any remaining malignant tissue.

The authors concluded their report with an appeal for more research on the effects of high-dosage CoQ_{10} for cancer patients.

Five Reasons to Consider CoQ_{10} in Cancer Therapy

It makes sense to consider the use of CoQ_{10} supplementation as part of an overall anticancer strategy for five principal reasons:

1. It is a major antioxidant, that is, it combats the free radical activity that is involved in the development of degenerative diseases, including cancer.

2. Chemotherapy increases free radical activity and impairs the immune system. For instance, *Adriamycin,* one widely used chemotherapy drug, apparently contributes to cardiac toxicity by generating overwhelming oxidative stress in the heart muscle cells, as well as inhibiting CoQ_{10}-dependent enzymes. A series of small studies have shown that CoQ_{10} supplementation can help prevent the poisoning of the heart without interfering with the antitumor effects of the drug.

3. Studies indicate that CoQ_{10} can increase the immune system's "firepower" against disease.

4. The body's natural CoQ_{10} level decreases with age, and animal studies show that the immune system's effectiveness also decreases in the presence of lower CoQ_{10}.

5. Most malignancies occur in the elderly, who have lowered immune response.

Gian Paolo Littarru, M.D., a leading CoQ_{10} researcher for thirty years, is presently directing medical investigations on the cancer-CoQ_{10} connection in Italy, where he is professor of medical chemistry at the University of Ancona.

"Our research has a two-fold purpose," he says. "First, we want a better understanding of CoQ_{10}'s anti-cancer potential and to see if it strengthens the effect of conventional therapy. And second, we want to know if administration of CoQ_{10} minimizes the side effects of the potent anti-cancer drugs."

In recent years, the medical profession has become increasingly open to alternative treatments. Given the central role that CoQ_{10} plays in the body, it seems like too important a compound to ignore in the fight against a devastating disease such as cancer where conventional therapies have a poor track record for success.

CoQ_{10} and AIDS

HIV patients often have nutritional deficiencies, points out Littarru, and as a result "probably produce less CoQ_{10} because their bodies lack certain nutrient factors essential to make CoQ_{10}."

What is AIDS?
Acquired immune deficiency syndrome refers to a contagious viral condition (attributed to the HIV virus) that weakens the immune system, leaving the body vulnerable to different kinds of infections.

Indeed, very low levels have been found in AIDS patients. This was first determined in 1988 by Karl Folkers and colleagues at the Institute of Biomedical Research in Austin. Individuals with ARC (AIDS-related complex), where the HIV virus is present but no symptoms are in evidence, were deficient in CoQ_{10}, too, but not to the same degree as in AIDS patients.

Protects against AZT

In one informal case report, CoQ_{10} alone was used to treat two individuals with ARC. "These patients were doing well five and six years after they started," reported Folkers in 1991. "This is extremely encouraging. They are healthy, working, and leading normal lives. The basis of this response, we feel, is that CoQ_{10} also benefits the immune system very positively."

More recent laboratory research in Europe has shown that CoQ_{10} protects disease-fighting lymphocyte cells from the lethal effects of the AIDS drug AZT.

To date, however, not enough research has been done to determine the extent of CoQ_{10}'s value against AIDS. Still, high-dosage CoQ_{10} supplementation (keeping close attention to blood levels to make sure the compound is being absorbed well) may benefit patients at any stage of the disease.

Chronic Fatigue

From a medical standpoint, supplementation with CoQ_{10} often generates considerable energy increases in patients who for some reason are energy depleted. Clinicians who routinely use CoQ_{10} in their practice say that it is well worth trying.

One such physician is Martin P. Gallagher, M.S., D.C., a nutritional therapy expert practicing in Jeannette, Pennsylvania. He consistently finds that CoQ_{10} elevates the energy of patients. "I see many patients with chronic fatigue syndrome who reach a certain plateau of improvement on a comprehensive healing program," he says.

"The program includes detoxification, a more nutritious diet, and supplementation with a broad array of important vitamins, minerals, and herbs. I usually reserve the CoQ_{10} for when a patient hits the plateau, and then, within two-to-six weeks of starting it, there is usually a discernible improvement in energy and strength."

Chronic fatigue syndrome typically has many causes. But physicians say that CoQ_{10} almost always helps reduce the fatigue level to some degree for as long as it is taken. Any energy gains will be lost if it is discontinued.

Prominent nutritional researcher Melvyn R. Werbach, M.D., writing in *Alternative Medicine Review,* includes a low level of CoQ_{10} among a list of key deficiencies that probably contribute to the syndrome and also stymie the healing process. Other pivotal deficiencies cited include the B vitamins, essential fatty acids, L-carnitine, magnesium, vitamin C, and zinc. Because of their therapeutic benefits, Werbach suggests supplementing chronic fatigue patients with these nutrients, along with a general high-potency vitamin and mineral formula.

CHAPTER 9

COMBATING NERVOUS SYSTEM DISORDERS

After starting CoQ_{10} supplementation, an eight-year-old boy confined to a wheelchair was able to walk independently, and a twenty-year-old woman was able to work outside the home for the first time.

These dramatic stories of recovery were recounted by Salvatore DiMauro, M.D., a neurologist and researcher at Columbia University in New York, in a 2001 issue of the journal *Neurology.*

DiMauro described two patients with hereditary ataxia, a rare incurable disorder that causes deterioration of the cerebellum, the part of the brain controlling coordination. Patients have difficulty with balance, coordination of arms and legs, and speech, and may develop seizures. DiMauro had discovered that the two patients, and four others with this condition he treated, had CoQ_{10} levels 70 percent lower than normal. He then began prescribing CoQ_{10} at daily dosages ranging from 300–3,000 mg.

Ataxia Patients Improved

"All of the patients improved," he reported. "They got stronger, their ataxia improved, and their seizures either stopped or happened less often." Five of the patients had been unable to walk before using CoQ_{10}. One year later, all were able to walk with some assistance, such as a rolling walker.

"Our findings suggest that CoQ_{10} deficiency is a potentially important cause of some forms of familial ataxia and it should be considered when diagnosing this condition," DiMauro said. "Where low levels are found, treatment to replace the missing

CoQ_{10} should be aggressive and begin early."

DiMauro's research is part of a recent surge of medical interest in CoQ_{10}'s potential against brain and neuromuscular disorders. In the last five years, scientific investigations in this area have skyrocketed.

A Growing Field of CoQ_{10} Research

Leading CoQ_{10} researchers like Karl Folkers and Gian Paolo Littarru began studying the compound's effect on muscular dystrophy (MD) more than twenty years ago. Brought to public attention by the telethons of comedian Jerry Lewis, MD is an umbrella term for a group of genetic diseases that progressively weaken and destroy muscles controlling movement. Some forms of the disease also affect the heart and other involuntary muscles.

The early research with CoQ_{10} demonstrated that it could help improve heart function in these patients. More recently, the potential of CoQ_{10} has expanded dynamically to include Alzheimer's disease, ataxia, Huntington's disease, Parkinson's disease, and certain conditions known as mitochondrial myopathies. The latter are disorders of the muscles caused by abnormalities in the mitochondria.

How CoQ_{10} Protects Neurons

Neurons are cells in the brain and the nervous system. Like other cells in the body, they get their energy from the mitochondria. Researchers think that the combination of oxidative damage and mutations in the mitochondria, and the resulting drop in energy output, contribute to so-called neurodegenerative disorders. In English, that means conditions that disturb and kill nerve tissue.

"Even subtle functional alterations in these essential cellular dynamos can lead to insidious pathological changes in neurons," one researcher wrote. No wonder, then, that researchers have begun looking seriously at CoQ_{10}.

Just how much potential does it have? The most

dramatic results so far have occurred among patients who, because of a genetic defect, have a reduced level of CoQ_{10}, a situation referred to as primary CoQ_{10} deficiency.

But even results where a primary deficiency is not involved are quite promising and have encouraged scientists to keep digging. Bioenergetic therapies, they say, may benefit the course of neurologic diseases in which mitochondrial function is impaired and oxidative stress and damage are present.

Huntington's Disease

Huntington's disease (HD) is a devastating, degenerative brain disorder without an effective treatment or cure. HD slowly diminishes the ability to reason, talk, think, and walk, and eventually causes total dependence on others for personal care. This condition is one of the more common genetic diseases. More than a quarter of a million Americans have it or are at risk of inheriting the disease.

In a major multi-medical-center study, a group of 347 patients with early-stage disease were randomly chosen to receive either CoQ_{10} (300 mg twice a day), an experimental drug, a combination of CoQ_{10} and the drug, or an inert placebo pill.

The results, published in 2001 in the journal *Neurology*, indicated that none of the treatment strategies significantly stopped the decline in functional capacity over a thirty-month period. However, the researchers did report "a trend toward slowing" the decline among the CoQ_{10} takers. There were also beneficial trends in secondary measures.

CoQ_{10} reportedly promoted a longer ability to handle daily responsibilities such as domestic chores and finances, a better ability to focus, and less depression and irritability.

"The First Real Lead"

The changes were not sufficient enough to allow the researchers to recommend CoQ_{10} for treatment of HD. Still, Karl Kieburtz, M.D., professor of neurology at the University of Rochester Medical Center, described the results as an "interesting lead" against a disease where there is currently no way to slow the progression. A bigger study was warranted, he said.

"This is the first real lead we've gotten from more than a dozen Huntington's disease patient trials," said Kieburtz. "We can't ignore it. We've got something to chase."

Mitochondrial Myopathies

Hundreds of varieties of these diseases have been identified. Symptoms include various degrees of deafness, diabetes, heart problems, learning disabilities, muscle weakness and cramps, paralysis of eye muscles, seizures, and strokelike episodes.

CoQ_{10} supplementation appears beneficial for myopathy patients who have few options. There is no cure, but research shows that CoQ_{10} helps reduce defective bioenegetics inside of cells, and helps improve muscle movement.

"In these patients, even what can be considered a small improvement by healthy peoples' standards actually represents a considerable achievement," says CoQ_{10} researcher Gian Paolo Littarru. "I have personally witnessed the heartwarming progress of some patients who are able to walk better or to climb three flights of stairs where they were barely able to make one flight before."

Brain Toxicity

Studies conducted by M. Flint Beal, M.D., a neurologist at Massachusetts General Hospital, show that CoQ_{10} helps protects brain tissue from a variety of nerve toxins. In laboratory experiments, such toxins create significantly less injury in animals who are supplemented.

Beal, along with Italian researchers, has also demonstrated that CoQ_{10} protects against "excitoxicity." This condition occurs when the energy level of nerve cells falls, leading to cell damage and death.

Parkinson's Disease

Who hasn't seen those heart-wrenching pictures of the former heavyweight champion Muhammad Ali, his hands shaking and his speech slurred. The great boxer, and more than a million other Americans, suffer from Parkinson's disease, a disorder that progressively destroys the central nervous system. The disease also causes rigidity of muscles and slowness of movement.

Parkinson's is believed to be caused by a combination of biochemical defects, including free radical damage and mitochondrial-DNA mutation, that destroy cells in the substantia nigra. This part of the brain produces dopamine, a chemical substance that enables people to move normally and smoothly. In Parkinson's, there is a severe shortage of dopamine.

Researchers know that brain tissue is highly susceptible to free radical damage. They also know that the substantia nigra has the highest level of mitochondrial-DNA mutation in the brain. These events conspire to harm cellular energy production. Researchers now believe that energy consumption plays a large role in the progression of the disease.

CoQ_{10} Studies Promising

Beal and his research colleagues at Massachusetts General Hospital have conducted a fascinating series of revealing studies on CoQ_{10} and Parkinson's. They found that the bioenergetic reduction in patients is strongly associated with the patients' blood levels of CoQ_{10}.

They also determined that CoQ_{10} supplementation could significantly reduce the amount of damage in the dopamine system of mice treated with a neurotoxin causing symptoms similar to Parkinson's.

And, in both human patients and mice, they found that supplementation helps restore sluggish energy production in the mitochondria. For humans, they found that 600 mg was an effective dose.

In a follow-up study sponsored by the National Institute of Neurological Disorders and Stroke, researchers compared daily dosages of 300, 600, and 1200 mg on patients with early Parkinson's who as yet did not require medication. The results of this study are due in 2002 and will further clarify the extent of effectiveness and dose tolerance of CoQ_{10} supplementation.

Alzheimer's Disease

Even when the health of former presidents like Ronald Reagan is involved, the big guns of mainstream medicine have woefully little firepower to use against the relentless loss of mental faculties and function caused by Alzheimer's disease (AD).

What is Alzheimer's disease?
Alzheimer's disease is currently the most common form of dementia illnesses. It causes progressive impairment of behavior, memory, and thinking, eventually leaving its victims unable to care for themselves.

There is no definitive cure. No definitive treatment. No definitive explanation of causes. AD affects about 10 percent of Americans over age sixty-five and nearly 50 percent of those over age eighty-five. Four million or more Americans now have AD. Within decades, as the baby boomer generation ages, the numbers are expected to soar to about 14 million.

No one knows if AD has one underlying cause or many. Scientists have investigated biochemical deficiencies; bioenergetic deficits; free radical damage; genetic abnormalities; malfunctions in the body's defenses; toxicity from metals such as aluminum, lead, and mercury; and viruses. Some researchers talk in terms of a "deleterious network" of events that causes AD to develop and progress.

More CoQ$_{10}$ Research Needed

There is no direct research on supplementation with CoQ$_{10}$ for Alzheimer's, except for one small Japanese study reported in a 1992 issue of the medical journal *Lancet*. In that study, 60 mg of CoQ$_{10}$ daily, along with vitamin B$_6$ and iron, was shown to slow down the progression of the disease.

Recent studies have linked the degree of disability in patients with a decline of energy production and mitochondrial efficiency in brain cells. This suggests a possible CoQ$_{10}$ role.

Scientists have cited the complicity of certain toxic proteins and free radicals in the damage and death of brain cells that occurs in AD. A byproduct of this activity is a toxin called HNE, which is found in excess amounts throughout the AD-affected brain. CoQ$_{10}$ and vitamin E, both antioxidants, have been shown to reduce HNE formation in the bloodstream.

Research Should Include Other Supplements

At this point, little can be said about CoQ$_{10}$ and Alzheimer's except that research is certainly warranted, and probably should include both CoQ$_{10}$ and vitamin E. Vitamin E has also been found to slow down progression of the disease.

It is worth mentioning that studies continually find the aging population suffering from malnutrition, failing to get proper amounts of nutrients because of altered gastrointestinal function, imbalances in food or diet, malabsorption, or multiple drug use. And patients with dementia and AD are more likely to be nutritionally deficient than healthy older people.

Thus, a comprehensive nutritional-supplement package should be investigated for effectiveness against Alzheimer's. Included in it should be therapeutic dosages of CoQ$_{10}$ and vitamin E, along with fatty acids, the B-complex vitamins, and other cellular "energizers," such as the amino acid L-carnitine. And, ideally, such a nutritional "cocktail" should be administered at the very earliest stage of the disease in an effort to slow down its progression.

Amyotrophic Lateral Sclerosis— "Lou Gehrig's Disease"

This devastating disease, which cut short the baseball career and life of famed New York Yankee great Lou Gehrig, attacks the nerves cells responsible for muscle control, causing loss of muscle function and paralysis. The cause of ALS is not completely understood and there is no cure. Some 5,000 Americans are diagnosed with this condition each year.

Researchers at Columbia-Presbyterian Medical Center's Eleanor and Lou Gehrig ALS Center in New York have begun investigating a possible therapeutic role for CoQ_{10}.

Promising Pilot Study on ALS

In a small pilot study completed in 2001, the center announced that high-dose CoQ_{10} supplementation had resulted in "positive trends." This development encouraged the center to set up a larger trial, which is underway.

In the pilot study, lasting nine months, six patients took 600 mg of CoQ_{10} daily. At the end of that period, researchers determined that the supplement could be beneficial for preserving motor units. A motor unit consists of a muscle-controlling nerve cell and the muscle cells it controls. A patient with ALS typically loses about 50 percent of existing motor units over a six-month period. With CoQ_{10}, three patients actually showed minimal *gains* in motor-unit numbers, while the other three had losses of 16, 23, and 38 percent.

Due to the small number of patients, the researchers were reluctant to draw conclusions from the pilot study, but felt the positive trend strongly justified a follow-up study. Enrollment for the bigger study began in October 2001.

CHAPTER 10

KEEPING YOUR
GUMS HEALTHY

Most people develop gum disease at some point in their adult life and unless they take care of the problem, it's bye-bye teeth. Gum disease (also called periodontal disease or periodontitis) is the leading cause of tooth loss.

Gum disease is usually treated by specialists who perform gum surgery or extract loose teeth. These specialists are known as periodontists. Some dentists also use non-surgical methods to treat periodontal disease, including a wide variety of nutritional supplements. High on their list of supplements is CoQ_{10}.

The dental use of CoQ_{10} dates back to the 1970s when researchers in Europe and Japan found a common deficiency among many patients with diseased gums. Further research showed that supplementation had a beneficial therapeutic effect.

In one double-blind clinical experiment over a three-week period, a group of patients were given either a placebo or a pill with 50 mg of CoQ_{10}. All eight patients on CoQ_{10} improved significantly. The placebo group showed no improvement.

Gum Disease

Problems start with gingivitis, an inflammation of the gums resulting from bacterial plaque formation. The bacteria eat away the supportive gum tissue of the teeth. Untreated gingivitis becomes periodontitis, with progressive infection, inflammation, deepening pockets between the gums and teeth, and the development of bone recession and loose teeth.

The CoQ_{10} patients had less pain, swelling, bleeding, and looseness of teeth, and reduced gingival pocket depth. CoQ_{10} also helped accelerate healing. The researchers said the results seen after three weeks of supplementation would normally take six months of treatment.

In Miami, Steven Green, D.D.S., has used CoQ_{10} for years. He regards it as a remarkable agent to counteract "fatigued" gum tissue. "At the most basic level there is no disease, including gum disease, that strikes anyone unless there is fatigue," he says. "CoQ_{10} is great for fatigue, because it enhances energy inside the mitochondria."

In the early 1980s, Green started using a 1-mg capsule (the only potency that was commercially available at the time), but did not see any clinical benefits. The dosage simply wasn't high enough. In time, CoQ_{10} capsules in 10-mg strength became available. He then recommended two capsules a day to ten patients on two-month recall. That means their periodontal disease was very advanced and they needed to be seen every other month.

"Their situations were so precarious that we would discuss at each visit whether it was time for them to bite the bullet and go for surgery," Green recalls. "They had all the classical symptoms that called for more invasive treatment—deep pockets, easily bleeding gums, rapid formation of plaque, and general tenderness of the gums. But they refused to see a specialist. They preferred to stick with the non-surgical approach. And even though I had been able to help them hold their own, I hadn't been able to make any headway."

Dramatic Improvement

"As these CoQ_{10} patients started returning, I checked for results. In six out of the ten cases, improvement was dramatic: two- and three-millimeter shrinkage of pockets. I had never seen anything work like that, and so fast. There was also significantly less bleeding."

Except for adding CoQ$_{10}$, the six patients had made no other changes. The other four patients who took CoQ$_{10}$ showed no such improvement. Still, the results encouraged Green to continue using CoQ$_{10}$ on a regular basis.

Craig Zunka, D.D.S., of Front Royal, Virginia, says he often reserves CoQ$_{10}$ as the "big cannon" in resistant cases. "Because CoQ$_{10}$ is expensive, I tend to use other supplements first," he says. "Initially, I will use antioxidants such as vitamin C and E and bring in CoQ$_{10}$ when I don't see the desired results."

Reduces Pockets and Bleeding

From Zunka's observations, CoQ$_{10}$ helps reduce bleeding and improve the texture and health of the gum tissue. Polly Hoverter, a dental hygienist in Zunka's office, describes how CoQ$_{10}$ dramatically helped to restore one patient with moderate-to-severe disease.

"This woman came in with many five- to six-millimeter pockets," says Hoverter. Within three months, all the pockets were down to three millimeters. Within six months, most had shrunk down to two millimeters. Her gums, previously bleeding and with an unhealthy grayish tint, were now pink and healthy-looking. The CoQ$_{10}$ really seemed to have helped her gums get healthy from the inside out."

Clean Pockets First, Then Use CoQ$_{10}$

Depending on what blood chemistries and other tests reveal, holistic dentists carefully individualize the array of supplements they recommend to gum-disease patients. These supplements are pivotal in the non-surgical treatment of gum disease.

"We need first of all to clean up the deep pockets between the gum and the tooth, deep down, where your brushing and flossing can't reach," says Zunka.

"It is this deep-down clearing of the bacteria that is the critical element. We then irrigate the depths of that pocket with a wide variety of natural herbal and nutritional solutions. We train our patients how to use irrigation tools on their own at home so they can become an active part of the healing process.

"Some people don't need any supplements, or just a few," adds Zunka. "They just need all the bacteria and tartar cleaned out and then their bodies will do the rest. Others need to have their immune system and cellular energetics pushed to the max with all the supplements you can throw at them."

CoQ_{10} Is Part of an Aggressive Nutritional Approach

In Manchester, Connecticut, periodontist Salvatore J. Squatrito, Jr., D.D.S., uses CoQ_{10} as part of an aggressive nutritional approach to improve the gum health of patients.

"In order to get good healing, patients need to eat a better diet, with five to seven fruits and vegetables a day and twelve glasses of water, and they need to minimize their intake of sugar, carbonated drinks, and alcohol," he says. "And because of the way food is grown and processed today, supplementation is a necessity."

Squatrito has been recommending CoQ_{10} for nearly ten years. "Patients who stick with it have less long-range trouble than they did in the past, before I used CoQ_{10}," he says. There is less bleeding and a gradual improvement in periodontal health.

Particularly Effective for Advanced Cases

CoQ_{10} is particularly beneficial for patients with "refractory disease." This refers to advanced cases that do not respond well to therapy. They are characterized by major pockets, pus, and inherited genetic weakness in the gums.

"These factors are indicative of low resistance," says Squatrito. "I place these patients on CoQ_{10} and a low-potency antibiotic to clear up the bacterial infections. Diet scans usually turn up nutritional deficiencies, so I recommend a whole range of other supplements as well to help build up resistance. We monitor diet very closely and do a lot of nutritional counseling with these patients in order to get results.

"The nature of their condition requires more effort, and more elbow grease on their part, to overcome it. "CoQ$_{10}$ is not a panacea. You have to limit the hostile environment. That means shrinking the pockets. You have to strengthen the patient at the same time. Then the chances of recurrence are minimized. But if you have deep pockets, and you only load up with CoQ$_{10}$ and think you will be OK, it won't happen."

The Risk of Spreading Infection

Squatrito says that a detailed periodontal charting and pocket-depth reading is necessary. Pockets deeper than four or five millimeters must be treated professionally. If not treated, they will accumulate hostile bacteria and the periodontal infection will advance.

"The risk is not just losing teeth," he says. "The infection can seep into your system, sap your energy, and even attack your heart."

Squatrito recommends that patients obtain a blood test to determine their CoQ$_{10}$ level. Such a test may or may not be covered by insurance, and will have to be done through a physician.

"From my experience, if the blood level is not over 2.5 micrograms of CoQ$_{10}$ per milliliter of blood, the likelihood of periodontal disease and recurrent infection is high," he says. "I try to have patients take enough CoQ$_{10}$ bring them up to a 2.5 or 3 microgram level. That's what can make a difference.

"I might start patients with 60 milligrams in the morning and another 60 milligrams in the evening, and see what kind of response they get. When I recheck them, and I find that the gingival fluid is cloudy, then I know they need more CoQ$_{10}$ and should probably be on an antibiotic as well.

"I am often able to get patients to the point where I only see them every six months or a year, and then I have little to do. That's a whole lot better for patients than having to return every two months, getting reamed out and having their gums drained."

The Patient Who Benefited Despite Himself

The great thing about CoQ_{10} is that it also does so many other good things for the body, dentists note. As an example, Squatrito cites a patient who "doesn't give a damn about his teeth," but without CoQ_{10} he can't walk up and down the steps without leg cramps. "That's why he takes it. It's the only reason. And it helps his teeth whether he's interested or not."

Dentists familiar with CoQ_{10} recommend taking 30–60 mg daily for prevention.

CHAPTER 11

How to Take
CoQ_{10}

Before we get into specifics, keep in mind that although CoQ_{10} can do wonders, it is not a panacea. Don't expect it to serve as a rescue remedy for every physical ailment or for a ruinous lifestyle.

It is also important to point out that people with CoQ_{10} deficiencies often have deficiencies in other key nutrients that can contribute to ill health or poor healing. This is particularly true of older individuals and those with medical conditions taking pharmaceutical drugs, but nutritional surveys consistently show that Americans of all ages are deficient in many vital nutrients.

In view of this, it is probably in the best interest of overall good health to take CoQ_{10} along with a high-quality multivitamin and mineral formula, at the very least.

How Much to Take for Disease Prevention

Unlike many vitamins and minerals, CoQ_{10} is not considered an essential nutrient that we must obtain in our diets or perish. That's because we make CoQ_{10} in our bodies. And even though we may become deficient in CoQ_{10}, as a result of the aging process, certain genetic conditions, poor diet, stress, or the use of particular medications, the medical community is not yet advising supplementation for prevention.

Research on CoQ_{10} is extensive and increasing all the time, but no one really knows precisely what represents an ideal "preventive" dose of CoQ_{10}. The research on this has not yet been done, so at this point we need to rely on the CoQ$_{10}$ experts, the researchers and clinicians most familiar with it.

Take 30 to 100 Mg for General Health

One obvious expert is Texas cardiologist Peter Langsjoen who has himself been taking CoQ$_{10}$ and recommending it to patients for twenty years. He believes that a healthy person in their forties could probably take 30 or 60 mg a day and see a variety of benefits.

"What we know is for illness," he says. "You see measurable changes in blood levels and heart function somewhere between thirty and sixty milligrams a day. It would seem reasonable to take that much for general health purposes and energy."

Langsjoen takes 100 mg twice a day. "I'm forty-seven, a very busy practitioner, and in good health," he says. "I feel it gives me great energy."

To Help Prevent Heart Attacks

Fellow cardiologist Stephen Sinatra believes that CoQ$_{10}$ can help both young and old. He recommends a preventive dose of 100 mg daily.

"If you are older and tired, double that amount," he says. As a supplement to help prevent heart attacks, he suggests 100 or 200 mg a day, along with natural vitamin E (200 IU for women and 200 to 400 IU for men).

"Be sure to use a form of vitamin E that contains not just alpha tocopherol, the most common form, but also gamma tocopherol," he adds. "This form is more expensive but it is also more protective. Take at least twenty-five international units of gamma tocopherol."

"I strongly believe CoQ$_{10}$ helps prevent cancer," says Sinatra. "There are no controlled studies, but from what we know of blood levels in patients with cancer, I don't have reservations about younger people taking CoQ$_{10}$."

Over Fifty? Take CoQ$_{10}$ for the Rest of Your Life

Australian expert on aging and CoQ$_{10}$ Anthony Linnane, age seventy, believes that "everyone over fifty should take CoQ$_{10}$ for the rest of their life."

He also recommends 100 mg a day, and takes 500 mg a day himself. "You should also take plenty of vitamins C and E for their additional antioxidant benefits," he says. "We aren't perfect machines, so there is no reason we can't give our normal processes a bit of nutritional help from the outside and improve them."

How Much to Take for Therapeutic Effect

Therapeutic doses generally range from 100–600 mg a day.

Langsjoen recommends at least 100 mg to his heart patients for general therapeutic purposes.

"If you can afford it, take 100 milligrams twice a day," he says. "And people who are very sick should take 400 milligrams. I have used even more in some cases. People may need the higher doses if they don't absorb it well, or if they have substantial heart failure and a lot of edema."

Subjectively, how can you tell if the CoQ$_{10}$ you are taking is working for you? "The most obvious thing you'll notice is improved energy and stamina," says Langsjoen.

If Possible, Have Your Blood Level Checked

Objectively, you can ask your physician to conduct a blood test that measures CoQ$_{10}$. More and more medical laboratories are offering this service as interest in CoQ$_{10}$ rises. And with this development comes more accurate and reliable tests.

A normal blood level is .8 to 1.2 micrograms per milliliter of blood. However, to obtain therapeutic benefits, the experts say the level must be driven up into the 2.5 to 3.5 range through sustained supplementation.

Cardiologist Stephen Sinatra notes that CoQ$_{10}$ has occasionally failed to show therapeutic potency in medical studies because researchers weren't getting high enough blood levels due to inadequate doses being administered to those in the study. "I find that the higher the blood level of CoQ$_{10}$ in very elderly or sicker patients, the greater the benefits," he says.

Other Key Supplements May Be Necessary

"However, about 15 percent of my cardiac patients do not experience therapeutic improvements with CoQ$_{10}$ supplementation, even when I raise their blood levels to 3.5 micrograms," he adds.

"The CoQ$_{10}$ is indeed getting into the body but is just not enough on its own to achieve the desired results. In those cases, I add other key supplements, such as L-Carnitine and NADH."

Among nutritional supplements, CoQ$_{10}$ is relatively expensive. Capsules typically come in 10, 30, 50, 60, or 100 mg. A bottle of sixty 10-mg capsules may retail for around $7; a bottle of sixty 100-mg capsules for about $45.

You May Require Less Medication

If you are under a doctor's care, please consult with your physician before starting CoQ$_{10}$. As we've seen throughout this book, CoQ$_{10}$ has the ability to improve cellular energy and thus have a positive impact on many symptoms. The effects can be very striking.

For instance, it can lower high blood pressure. And if you take a significant dose of blood-pressure medication, you may become lightheaded because your pressure drops as a result of CoQ$_{10}$.

It is indeed probable that some medications can be reduced or somehow adjusted after CoQ$_{10}$ is started. This is generally desirable since drugs typically cause side effects and disturb normal processes in the body. But don't stop or reduce medication on your own. That should be done only under the guidance of a physician.

Your doctor may not know about CoQ_{10} or may dismiss it. In either case, you may want to show him or her this book and mention that there have been thousands of scientific studies proving CoQ_{10}'s effectiveness and safety. Keep in mind also that your doctor may have a bias against a simple nutritional supplement that he or she is not familiar with.

How to Take CoQ$_{10}$

If you slug down your vitamins with a glass of water whenever you remember, it is very probable you aren't getting a big bang for your CoQ_{10} buck. It works better if you take it with a meal, and preferably with a meal that has some fat in it. CoQ_{10} is a fat-soluble compound. That means it dissolves, and absorbs, more effectively in a fatty environment.

There is also a saturation effect with CoQ_{10}. Research shows that your body can only make use of about 180 mg maximum at a time, so if you take more in a single dose, you may not be utilizing the excess. If you take more than that amount, divide your daily dosage. "Most of my cardiac patients take it twice a day," says Langsjoen.

"To get the big heart benefits and other improvements, sick people need to take CoQ_{10} in big enough doses and with their food. Those are the two biggest mistakes when you don't see results: using Mickey-Mouse doses or not taking it with food."

Experts advise keeping CoQ_{10} away from heat and out of direct sunlight, so keep it stored in a cool, dark pantry, for instance.

How Safe Is CoQ$_{10}$?

CoQ_{10} is extremely safe to take. I've never heard of anything in the way of complaints in any shape, form, or fashion," says Langsjoen. "And I have prescribed

CoQ_{10} to thousands of patients." The medical literature mentions 1 or 2 percent of users experiencing some upset stomach. "But I have never come across this or any other effect in nearly twenty years of using CoQ_{10}," Langsjoen adds. If an upset stomach develops, try reducing the amount of CoQ_{10} you take, or switch to a different form (see the section below on forms of CoQ_{10}).

One recent Scandinavian report stated that the effectiveness of coumadin, a commonly prescribed blood thinner, was decreased in three patients who took CoQ_{10}. Langsjoen has specifically looked for this effect and has never observed it, even using amounts much greater than those used in the Scandinavian cases.

Are All Forms of CoQ₁₀ Equal?

Although the original discoveries of CoQ_{10} occurred in the United States, Japan has dominated the commercial production. In the mid-1970s, the fermentation technology that produces pure CoQ_{10} from yeast was developed there. Today, two Japanese pharmaceutical companies supply most of the CoQ_{10} used in supplements and medical research. Quality is quite good, say the experts.

Supplements are commonly found in three forms: as capsules containing yellow powder, soft-gels with CoQ_{10} dissolved in a natural oil base, or tablets. If you don't see the expected results from one form of CoQ_{10}, you may want to switch to another. It could be you are not absorbing that particular supplement well.

"When you treat people with CoQ_{10} and they don't react to the compound, they are probably not absorbing it," says cardiologist Stephen Sinatra. "I have seen patients taking as much as 500 milligrams daily, yet they have an ordinary blood level that they might have from just their regular diet.

"I saw a young man with cardiomyopathy who was taking 200 milligrams a day and yet his blood level was .8 micrograms. I put him on a different form of CoQ_{10} which elevated his blood level up to 3.5 micrograms, and he had a totally different quality of life."

Langsjoen contends that "no matter what kind of CoQ_{10} you take, you can get just about a doubling of the blood level by swallowing it with a meal as opposed to taking it with water alone. That alone makes a big difference."

The Vitamin B_6 Connection

The B-complex vitamins, and particularly B_6, are key ingredients used by certain enzymes in the body to produce CoQ_{10}. Both vitamin B_6 and CoQ_{10} levels decline as we age. For that reason, researchers at the University of Texas in Austin recommended that patients receiving supplemental CoQ_{10} also be supplemented with vitamin B_6. That would enhance better synthesis of CoQ_{10} in the body to go along with the supplement, they wrote in a 1999 report in the journal *Biofactors*.

As noted, CoQ_{10} is relatively expensive. Thus, individuals who cannot afford the higher therapeutic doses may want to boost their own CoQ_{10} production with a B_6 supplement. B_6 is inexpensive.

Peter Langsjoen relates the case of a patient with very low levels of B_6 and CoQ_{10}. The patient couldn't easily afford CoQ_{10}, but was readily able to purchase the vitamin. "I suggested 100 milligrams of B_6 a day," recalls Langsjoen. "I rechecked his CoQ_{10} level in about two months, and it had significantly increased. The level wasn't as high as the therapeutic dose of CoQ_{10} I felt he needed, but I was impressed by the increase created by B_6. And his B_6 level was now normal."

CHAPTER 12

THE FUTURE
OF CoQ$_{10}$

Modern medicine has taken the approach that a disease can be furiously and selectively attacked with the likes of antibiotics, powerful drugs, chemotherapy, and surgery, without any damage to the host body. It's a medical myth.

Someone may be cured of one condition only to suffer or die from something else caused by the treatment. In general, the time borrowed with medication and surgery does not mean that health has been restored.

Patients are demanding a change. And as our medical system matures, it will likely come to honor the need to strengthen the body with key nutritional supplements such as CoQ$_{10}$. This is what an integrative medical approach is all about, and today many large hospitals and major university medical centers have taken steps in this direction by opening "complementary" or "alternative" clinics.

The Changing Medical Scene

In this shifting ambiance, interested patients should have more access to savvy doctors who believe in and use many natural healing remedies. Such practitioners may recommend a certain drug and a nutritional supplement to prevent side effects and bolster the body from the onslaught of drug or surgical stress. The idea is really to use the best combination of approaches, not just one that takes away the symptom and leaves the cause of the disease still smoldering in the body.

CoQ$_{10}$ is not a patented drug. It's a natural compound. You can't patent it. And because of this, it has no big pharmaceutical sugar daddy pushing major research, advertising in medical journals, peddling it to doctors, and staging media blitzes. This is why it has taken decades to get the word out. But CoQ_{10} is just too good for researchers and doctors to ignore.

The late Karl Folkers, the respected University of Texas researcher who studied CoQ_{10} for decades, believed that the supplement had huge medical applications, from brain disorders to cancer to heart disease. "When you favorably affect the bioenergetics of your cells, the results show up in all tissues," he said.

Even a Small Deficiency Could Be Critical

As medical science probes deeper into the mitochondrial and bioenergetic basis for disease and the aging process itself, CoQ_{10} figures to keep gaining more importance. Rolf Luft, M.D., Ph.D., of the Karolinska Hospital in Sweden, and one of the pioneers in mitochondrial medicine, has observed that even a relatively small deficiency of CoQ_{10} may be a key factor in the development of mitochondrial disorders.

Mitochondrial medicine is a dynamic frontier of current research. Some scientists refer to it as a revolution in medical and aging research. And the results of 4,000 studies already make it clear that we have a uniquely powerful healing and protective friend in CoQ_{10}.

Researchers in Europe even think that CoQ_{10} may reduce the detrimental oxidation of skin tissue that contributes to wrinkling and aging skin. Thus, you can now buy skin creams containing CoQ_{10}.

And recently, Italian researchers found that patients with macular degeneration, the leading cause of blindness in people older than fifty, have low levels of CoQ_{10}. They believe that CoQ_{10} may be able to help counteract the free radical damage thought to be the basis of this age-associated disease.

An Exciting Future

CoQ$_{10}$ has gained increasing attention simply because it plays a very central role in the body. Can you name a single drug with so many healing benefits? And can you name any drug that does so much without any side effects?

Many practitioners of nutritional medicine have long used CoQ$_{10}$ as part of their treatment strategies. Often, they use it as part of a multiple antioxidant combination (along with such nutrients as alpha-lipoic acid, l-carnitine, and vitamins A, C, and E) to generate a broad-spectrum healing effect.

But whether alone or in combination, CoQ$_{10}$ clearly represents a major weapon for doctors in their battle against disease. Hopefully, they will recognize it and use it because ignoring it is a major disservice to patients.

Fred Crane, the research biochemist who started it all with his discovery of CoQ$_{10}$ back in 1957, sums it up when he says, "what we do know about CoQ$_{10}$ is very exciting . . . and what we still don't know figures to be even more exciting."

SELECTED
REFERENCES

Baggio, E, et al. Italian multicenter study on safety and efficacy of coenzyme Q_{10}. *The Molecular Aspects of Medicine*, 1994; 15:S287–S294.

Blasi, MA, Bovina, C, Carella, G, et al. Does coenzyme Q_{10} play a role in opposing oxidative stress in patients with age-related macular degeneration? *Ophthalmologica*, 2001; 215(1):51–54.

Bliznakov, E, Casey, A, Premuzic, E. Coenzyme Q: Stimulants of the phagocytic activity in rats and immune response in mice. *Experientia*, 1970; 26:953–54.

Folkers, K, Brown, R, Judy, W, et al. Survival of cancer patients on therapy with coenzyme Q_{10}. *Biochemical and Biophysical Research Communication*, April 15, 1993; 192(1):241–245.

Folkers, K, Langsjoen, P, Willis, R, et al. Lovastatin decreases coenzyme Q levels in humans. *Proceedings of the National Academy of Sciences*, 1990; 87:8931–8934.

Folkers, K, Wolaniuk, J, Simonsen, R, et al. Biochemical rationale and the cardiac response of patients with muscle disease to therapy with coenzyme Q_{10}. *Proceedings of the National Academy of Sciences*, 1985; 82: 4513–4516.

Hoppe, U. Coenzyme Q_{10}: a cutaneous antioxidant and energizer. Presented at the First Conference of the International Coenzyme Q_{10} Association, 1998.

Iwamoto, Y, Watanabe, T, Okamoto, H, et al. Clinical effect of coenzyme Q_{10} on periodontal disease. In: Folkers, K, Yamamura, Y, (eds) *Biomedical and Clinical Aspects of Coenzyme Q_{10}*, Elsevier, Amsterdam, 1981; vol.3:109–119.

Langsjoen, P, Langsjoen, PH, Treatment of essential hypertension with coenzyme Q_{10}. *Molecular Aspects of Medicine*, 1994; 15supplement:S265–S272.

Langsjoen, PH, Langsjoen, AM. Overview of the use of CoQ_{10} in cardiovascular disease. *Biofactors*, 1999; 9 (2–4):273–284.

Linnane, AW, Marzuki, S, Ozawa, T, et al. Mitochondrial DNA mutations as an important contributor to ageing and degenerative diseases. *Lancet*, 1989; 1(8639): 642–645.

Linnane, A W, et al. Cellular redox activity of coenzyme Q_{10}: Effect of CoQ_{10} supplementation on human skeletal muscle. In press: *Free-Radical Research*, 2002.

Lockwood, K, Moesgaard, S, Folkers, K. Partial and complete regression of breast cancer in patients in relation to dosage of coenzyme Q_{10}. *Biochemical and Biophysical Research Communications*, 1994; 199(3): 1504–1508.

Lockwood, K, Moesgaard, S, Yamamoto, T, et al. Progress on therapy of breast cancer with vitamin Q_{10} and the regression of metastases. *Biochemical and Biophysical Research Communications*, 1995; 212:172–177.

Luft, R. The development of mitochondrial medicine. *Biochimica et Biophysica Acta*, May 24, 1995; 1271:1–6.

Mazzio, E, Huber, J, Darling, S, et al. Effect of antioxidants on L-glutamate and N-methyl-4-phenylpyridinium ion-induced neurotoxicity in PC12 cells. *Neurotoxicology*, April 2001; 22(2)283–8.

Musumeci, O, Hirano, M, DiMauro, S, et al. Familial cerebellar ataxia with muscle coenzyme Q_{10} deficiency. *Neurology*, April 2001; 56(7):849–855.

Pepe, S, Lyon, W, Rosenfeldt, FL, et al. Improved outcomes in coronary artery bypass graft surgery with preoperative coenzyme Q_{10} therapy: A randomized, double-blind placebo-controlled Trial. Presented at the 2001 American Heart Association Scientific Sessions Conference in Anaheim, CA.

Thomas, SR, Witting, PK, Stocker, R. A role for reduced coenzyme Q in atherosclerosis? *Biofactors*, 1999; 9 (2–4):207-224.

OTHER BOOKS AND RESOURCES

Bliznakov, Emile, and Hunt, Gerald. *The Coenzyme Q10 Phenomenon.* New York, NY: Bantam Books, 1987.

Littarru, Gian Paolo. *Energy and Defense: Facts and Perspectives on Coenzyme Q10 in Biology and Medicine.* Rome, Italy: Casa Editrice Scientifica Internazionale, 1995.

Sinatra, Stephen. *The Coenzyme Q10 Phenomenon.* Chicago, IL: Keats NTC/Contemporary Publishing Group, 1998.

Let's Live Magazine
Consumer magazine with emphasis on the health benefits of vitamins, minerals, and herbs.
Customer service:
1-800-676-4333
P.O. Box 74908
Los Angeles, CA 90004
Subscriptions: 12 issues per year, $19.95 in the U.S.; $31.95 outside the U.S.

Physical Magazine
Magazine oriented to body builders and other serious athletes.
Customer service:
1-800-676-4333
P.O. Box 74908
Los Angeles, CA 90004
Subscriptions: 12 issues per year, $19.95 in the U.S.; $31.95 outside the U.S.

The Nutrition Reporter™ newsletter
Monthly newsletter that summarizes recent medical research on vitamins, minerals, and herbs.

Customer service:
P.O. Box 30246
Tucson, AZ 85751-0246
e-mail: jack@thenutritionreporter.com
www.nutritionreporter.com
Subscriptions: $26 per year (12 issues) in the U.S.; $32 U.S. or $48 CNC for Canada; $38 for other countries

Coenzyme Q10 Association
www.coenzymeq10.org
A worldwide group of researchers and clinicians with a special interest in CoQ$_{10}$.

MEDLINE
http://www.ncbi.nlm.nih.gov/entrez/query
For specific medical journal abstracts.

INDEX

Printed in the USA
CPSIA information can be obtained
at www.ICGtesting.com
JSHW051956150824
68134JS00050B/52